Wolfgang Grimm
Stability Testing of Drug Products

Paperback APV

Die Buchreihe wird im Auftrag der Arbeitsgemeinschaft für Pharmazeutische Verfahrenstechnik e. V. (APV), Mainz, herausgegeben

Band 16

In der Reihe Paperback APV sind bereits erschienen:

Band 1 Hauschild
Ausgangsmaterialien für die Arz-
neimittelherstellung. Qualitätsanfor-
derungen (GMP) und deren Folgen für
Zulieferer und Pharma-Betriebe

Band 2 Essig/Schmidt/Stumpf
Flüssige Arzneimittelformen und Arz-
neimittelsicherheit. Unter besonderer Berücksichtigung der Qualität von Wasser

Band 3 Hasler
Dosierungsgenauigkeit einzeldosierter
fester Arzneiformen

Band 4 Brandau/Lippold
Dermal and Transdermal Absorption

Band 5 Schrank/Skinner
Arzneimittelhygiene von der Herstellung bis
zur Verabreichung

Band 6 Oeser
Selbstinspektion und Inspektion.
GMP-Forderungen zur Qualitätssicherung
im Arzneimittel-Bereich

Band 7 Fahrig/Hofer
Die Kapsel. Grundlagen, Technologie und
Biopharmazie einer modernen Arzneiform

Band 8 Sucker
Praxis der Validierung unter besonderer
Berücksichtigung der FIP-Richtlinien für
die gute Validierungspraxis

Band 9 Algner/Helbig/Spingler
Primär-Packmittel. Herstellung + Op-
timierung + Kontrolle = Sicherheit

Band 10 Asche/Essig/Schmidt
Technologie von Salben, Suspensionen und
Emulsionen

Band 11 Hanke
Qualität pflanzlicher Arzneimittel. Prüfung
und Herstellung – Anforderungen bei der
Zulassung

Band 12 Dertinger/Gänshirt/Steinigen
GAP – Praxisgerechtes Arbeiten in phar-
mazeutisch-analysierten Laboratorien

Band 13 Helbig/Singler
Kunststoffe für die Pharmazeutische
Verpackung. Einsatz – Anforderungen –
Prüfverfahren

Band 14 Brandau
Pharmaproduktion aus betriebswirtschaft-
licher Sicht

Band 15 Essig/Hofer/Schmidt/Stumpf
Stabilisierungstechnologie
Wege zur haltbaren Arzneiform

Band 17 Müller
Controlled Drug Delivery

Stability Testing of Drug Products

Scientific Criteries, guidelines and officiel state requirements in Europe, Japan and USA

Edited by Dr. Wolfgang Grimm,
Dr. Karl Thomae GmbH, D-Biberach

International APV Symposium
on Stability Testing of Pharmaceutical Products, (1985 : Munich)
Munich, December 2–4, 1985

Organized by
Dr. P. Fischer, CH-Bern
Prof. Dr. H. Feltkamp, Bayer AG, D-Leverkusen
Dr. W. Grimm, Dr. Karl Thomae GmbH, D-Biberach
Prof. Dr. H. Sucker, Sandoz AG, CH-Basel

with 104 figures and 8 tables

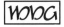

Wissenschaftliche Verlagsgesellschaft mbH Stuttgart 1987

Ein Markenzeichen kann warenzeichenrechtlich geschützt sein, auch wenn ein Hinweis auf etwa bestehende Schutzrechte fehlt.

CIP-Kurztitelaufnahme der Deutschen Bibliothek

Stability testing of drug products : scientif.
criteries, guidelines and official state requirements
in Europe, Japan and USA / Internat. APV Symposium
on Stability Testing of Pharmaceut. Products, Munich,
December 2–4, 1985. Ed. by Wolfgang Grimm. Organized
by P. Fischer ...– Stuttgart : Wissenschaftliche
Verlagsgesellschaft, 1987.
  (Paperback APV ; 16)
  ISBN 3-8047-0874-9
NE: Grimm, Wolfgang [Hrsg.]; International
Symposium on Stability Testing of Pharmaceutical
Products ‹1985, München›; International
Association for Pharmaceutical Technology:
Paperback APV

© 1987 Wissenschaftliche Verlagsgesellschaft mbH, Birkenwaldstraße 44, 7000 Stuttgart 1
Printed in Germany
Satz und Druck: Tutte Druckerei GmbH, 8391 Salzweg b. Passau
Umschlaggestaltung: Hans Hug, 7000 Stuttgart

Contents

XI. Stability and Stability Testing of Medicinal Products

Address of the authors:

Dr. W. Grimm,
Analytik,
Dr. Karl Thomae GmbH
Postfach 1755
D-7950 Biberach

Dr. M. Baltezor
Dorsey Laboratories
Box 83288
USA-Lincoln Nebraska 68501-3288

Prof. Dr. S. S. Davis,
Pharmacy Department,
University of Nottingham,
University Park,
Nottingham NG7 2Ra, UK

Prof. Dr. S. Ebel,
Faculty of Chemistry and Pharmacy
Department of Pharmaceutical
Chemistry,
University of Würzburg,
Am Hubland,
D-8700 Würzburg

Prof. Dr. G. Harnischfeger,
Schaper & Brümmer GmbH
Postfach 61 11 60
D-3320 Salzgitter 61

Prof. Dr. F. W. Hefendehl
Institut für Arzneimittel des
Bundesgesundheitsamtes
Seestraße 10
D-1000 Berlin 65

Dr. D. Herrmann,
Schering AG
D-1000 Berlin

Prof. Dr. R. Hüttenrauch,
VEB JENAPHARM,
Otto-Schott-Straße 13,
DDR-6900 Jena

B. Huyghe,
honoraise Inspecteur Général de la
Pharmacie
Ministère de la Santé Publique, Bruxelles,
Bosstraat 22,
B-2570 Duffel, Belgique

Dr. K. Krummen,
SANDOZ LTD.,
Basle, Switzerland

Professor Dr. T. Nagai,
Department of Pharmaceutics,
Hoshi University, Ebara,
Shinagawa-ku, Tokyo 142, Japan

Ap. Walter Oeser,
Alte Apotheke in Schnelsen
Frohmestraße 74
D-2000 Hamburg 61

Prof. Dr. F. Pellerin
Université Paris-Sud
Centre D'Études Pharmaceutiques
Les orntoire de Chemie Analytique
Rue Jean-Baptiste-Climent
F-92290 Châtenay-Malabry

Mr. Robert C. Shultz,
Division of Neuropharmacological
Drug Products,
Center for Drugs and Biologics,
Food and Drug Administration,
USA-Rockville, Maryland

Dr. A. G. Stewart
Department of Health and Social Security,
Market Tower 1 Nine Elms Lane,
GB-London SW8 5NQ

Prof. Dr. A. Verain et D. Chulia,
Université de Grenoble Faculté de
Pharmacie,
F-38240 Meylan Grenoble,
Avenue de Verdun

Introduction

The papers of this publication have been presented at the International Symposium on Stability Testing of Pharmaceutical Products in Munich, December 2–4, 1985, organized by the APV, the International Association for Pharmaceutical Technology. Prof. Dr. H. Feltkamp, Dr. P. Fischer, Dr. W. Grimm, Prof. Dr. Speiser and Prof. Dr. H. Sucker were responsible for the programme, the papers and the discussions.

The APV has already made several important contributions to the current state of knowledge and awareness of the problems of Stability Testing.

Specific examples include:
1972: APV Guidelines on Stability and Storage of Drugs
1974: GMP Symposium on Stability and Stability Testing in Hannover
1977: The first Course on Stability Testing of Pharmaceutical Preparations, which has since been repeated on twelve occasions with participants from 12 different countries.
1985: New revised and enlarged Guidelines on Stability and Stability Testing of Drugs.

These milestones illustrate the experience and competence of APV in this field and the intensive efforts the Association has made concerning drug stability, which have been continued in the International Symposium.

Stability Testing ensures that the perfect quality and hence the effectiveness of a drug product is maintained throughout its shelf life. It is therefore an important prerequisite of industrial drug manufacture.

The subject will be treated by scientists from Europe, Japan and the USA, representatives of the academic world, regulatory authorities and industry.

The authors describe the current state of technology, the crucial problems still to be solved, the direction in which stability testing should develop, so that future problems may be overcome.

Advances in pharmaceutical technology, biochemistry and medicine have shown that not only organoleptic criteria (appearance, smell, taste) and the content of active ingredient play an important role, but that stability testing must also include the examination of physicochemical, biochemical and microbiological parameters.

In future, questions will also arise from the area of biotechnology. Only when all the criteria of a drug relevant to stability are considered, can its effectiveness be ensured.

In the case of the technologically lavish dosage forms with their different depot principles, transdermal or even self-regulating systems, testing of the actual delivery concept can be even more important than merely measuring the content of drug.

Thus over the course of time, the demands on the Stability Test have risen quite markedly, have widened enormously in their scope and have long since escaped from the confines of a purely analytical science.

As a result of this broadening of the task and the shift in emphasis to physicochemical and biochemical criteria, a whole range of questions has emerged:

- How precise are the investigative methods used?
- How extensive are the changes that occur?
- How far can changes be tolerated?
- To what extent can changes be predicted?
- What is the cause of the changes?
- After what time may binding statements about stability be made?

These questions are addressed in the papers:

- Physicochemical changes from a molecular pharmaceutical point of view
- Physicochemical criteria for semisolid dosage forms
- Physicochemical criteria for solid dosage forms

Drugs are intended to cure, alleviate or prevent diseases. To what extent therefore, may stability-related changes be tolerated?

A reply to this question will be given from a medical viewpoint.

The need and purpose of Stability Tests are undisputed, however the precise outlay and scope necessary cannot be nearly so clearly answered.

This is also reflected in the various guidelines and draft guidelines of different countries on Stability and Stability Testing. Those of Japan, the USA, the EEC, the Federal Republic of Germany, France and Great Britain are presented here.

These national and international guidelines arose out of a desire to create a uniform standard of quality and were drawn up to assist manufactures in the execution of Stability Tests.

As however, the individual guidelines differ in their concepts, requirements and points of emphasis, difficulties arise if Stability Tests are undertaken for the registration of a drug product in different countries.

Two ways around this problem immediately come to mind:

- specific stability tests for each country
- one includes all the different requirements in a single Test.

Both solutions are unrealistic because,

- they require much too high an outlay

– They lead to a purely formalistic Stability Test directed not towards the particular problem, but to fulfil the various requirements.

Instead the aim should be to orientate Stability Tests along universally accepted principles which,

– take into account scientific knowledge
– match outlay and scope to the particular problem.

The APV Guidelines on Stability and Stability Testing offer a means of solving the problem.

Great progress has been made in the last few years in methods of analysis and analytical technology. Therefore the time is ripe to take stock of what has been achieved so far and at the same time to show to what extent the chromatographic techniques mostly used today will be replaced or supplemented in the future by alternative methods. In an attempt to obtain a uniform standard of quality for all drugs, the current position regarding the stability testing of phytopharmaceuticals and other natural substances and the methods employed in this area, will be described.

Industry has a wealth of experience in stability testing which can be drawn upon to show the effort and range of the investigations it carries out, their main focus of attention and purpose.

So the outlay which appears necessary for the practical execution of a Stability Test will be described.

So this book deals with the fundamental principles of the methods, execution and evaluation of Stability Tests and the scope of data on stability for drug registration, to enable

– Stability testing to provide its important contribution to drug safty,
– the execution and evaluation of results to be carried out on a scientific basis,
– Stability data to be mutually recognised in as many countries as possible.

Therefor this publication will be of great help for those from industry, regulatory bodies and universities who are themselves engaged in stability testing or the evaluation of stability data.

Wolfgang Grimm

I. Physico-chemical changes from a molecular-galenical viewpoint

R. Hüttenrauch, VEB Jenapharm, DDR-Jena

1. Introduction

Our life passes on under certain physical conditions, and it is only under these conditions that life is possible. The criteria include temperature, moisture, light and atmosphere (atmospheric oxygen). That is why the space within the boundaries of which terrestrial events proceed like in a cage has been referred to as "living-space or biosphere". Exceeding its limits will result in illness and death.

The conditions under which we live are the same for all things surrounding us and which we need for our existence to be based on. Among them are the medicinal drugs. Drugs, therefore, are subject to the same qualitive and quantitative influence as we ourselves are. And there are changes taking place in them like in an organism – they undergo ageing. The restriction of this "ageing process" would require a specific

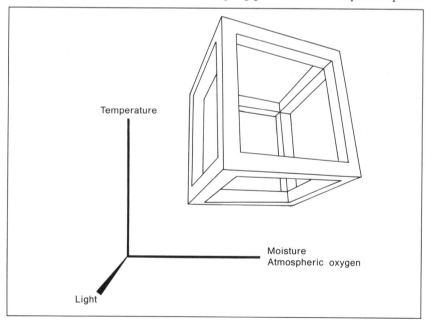

Fig. 1: Space of existence for people and drugs

Molecular Pharmaceutical Viewpoint

Physicochemical Changes = Changes in molecular DEGREE OF ORDER

3*Second Law* of Thermodynamics (R. Clausius)

All spontaneous (irreversible) processes always proceed so that the entropy (disorder) of the whole system increases,

$\Delta S > 0$

ΔS is the measure of the spontaneity (irreversibility, probability) of a process

---

Fig. 2: Order and disorder as decisive parameters of molecular pharmaceutics

protection of the drug. This measure, which is always a relative one, has been known as stabilization. We would have by far less stabilization trouble in a world, where very low temperatures, darkness and an inert gas atmosphere were prevalent.

To understand the causes of physicochemical changes occuring during a drug's storage requires that an approximately ten millionfold enlargement of the objects be used to look at them in their molecular structure, i. e. that molecular pharmaceutics be practised. The molecular-pharmaceutical view on the stabilization problems may be expressed as shown by Fig. 2 (1).

All phenomena should be taken as changes in the molecular state of order. And molecular order in thermodynamics being defined by the entropy, this variable is of major importance for drug stability considerations. Thus the first question is: in

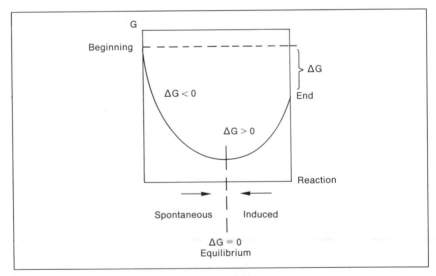

Fig. 3: Fundamental law of stability and instability

Eyring-Equation

$$\Delta G = -RT \cdot \ln K \qquad\qquad K \cdot v = k$$

$$K = e^{-\frac{\Delta G}{RT}} \qquad\qquad v = \frac{k_B T}{h}$$

$$\boxed{k = \frac{k_B T}{h} \, e^{-\frac{\Delta G}{RT}}} \quad = \frac{k_B T}{h} \, e^{-\frac{\Delta H}{RT}} \, e^{\frac{\Delta S}{R}}$$

$$-\Delta G = \left(\log \frac{k}{T} - \log \frac{k_B}{h} \right) 2,303 \, RT$$

$$-\Delta G = 5706 \log k - 72\,980 \qquad 25°C$$

Fig. 4: Dependence of the reaction rate upon driving force

which relation valid for all dosage forms and reaction types docs entropy characterize the tendency and direction of a system to change?

The molecules' "lives" and their behaviour towards one another are described by the GIBBS-HELMHOLTZ equation (Fig. 3).

In this formula the inner energy U and the free energy F have under isochoric conditions the same importance as have the enthalpy H and the free enthalpy G under the usual isobaric conditions. Of decisive weight for the driving force of a reaction (reactivity) is the difference of the free enthalpies between the final and initial states; this difference increases with the difference of the entropies. Hence the GIBBS-HELMHOLTZ equation is the formula looked for.

While storing a drug a spontaneous physicochemical change occurs, when the free enthalpy decreases during the process, i.e. the difference of the free enthalpies between final and initial states ($G_{afterwards}$ and G_{before}) assumes negative values. As soon as the thermodynamic equilibrium has been reached, this means, any further decrease of G is impossible and $\Delta G = O$, the process comes to a standstill. In this state only reversible processes take place such as are known to use in terms of a "dynamic equilibrium". Beyond the equilibrium, changes occur solely if forced, e. g. by the input of thermal energy. Thus definitions for stability and stabilization, which have not been usual in pharmacy as yet are derived from the GIBBS-HELMHOLTZ equation as follows:

The stability of a system is determined by the feasibility to reduce its free enthalpy. The driving force of each spontaneous process corresponds to the GIBBS free energy. A system behaves stable when the thermodynamic equilibrium has been reached and the difference of the free enthalpies between the final and initial states is zero. To stabilize means to realize or approach this equilibrium. The larger (less negative) is the difference between the free enthalpies the smaller is the rate of a process (EYRING equation). A process can also be inhibited or prevented by a reaction barrier (corresponding to an increased activation energy and equal to an inhibiting force).

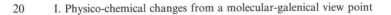

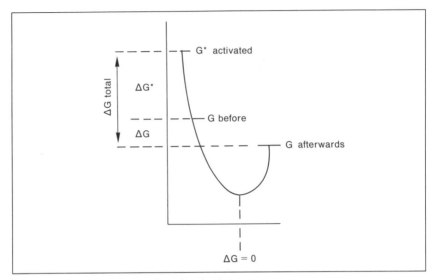

Fig. 5: Thermodynamic meaning of activation

This is the philosophy of stability. The conclusions result from the behaviour of the single molecules for each aggregate of molecules according to the principles of "Statistical Thermodynamics". The EYRING equation, which describes the connection of thermodynamics with kinetics, enables one to derive the reaction rate from the free enthalpies and, vice versa, the thermodynamic parameters from the kinetic ones (Fig. 4).

The process is directed by the second law of thermodynamics, which demands an increase of entropy (entropy production) in all spontaneous processes (see above).

When the free enthalpy of a system is increased by energy input, we call this

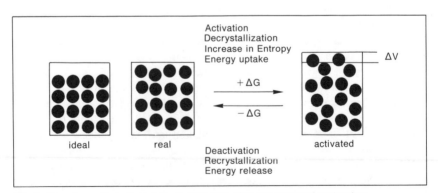

Fig. 6: Transformation of energy during and after mechanical activation

"activation". In this way also the GIBBS free energy and thus the driving force and rate of changes are enhanced, as if the molecules were given a reinforced swing by a greater run-up (Fig. 5).

Consequently, in pharmaceutics, too, it is conclusive for the stability set of problems, in how far there is an activated or an inactivated state present.

2. Solid and semi-solid dosage forms, solids in suspensions

Relating to solids besides the thermal also a mechanical activation is known, which is caused by friction or fracture and occurs, e.g. in the course of tabletting (Fig. 6).

The mechanically transferred energy is stored largely in the form of lattice defects by the solids, which, as a result, pass into a metastable state. A measure of the degree of activation consists in the so-called activation volume, which is comparable to the expansion volume in case of thermal activation. The activated systems having a tendency, while subject to inactivation and recrystallization, to re-release the excess energy input, chemical and physical reactions can thus be induced or enhanced (2). Such a phenomenon might be expected to occur in tablets. Due to the increase of ΔG agents in the tabletted state ought to behave less stable than in the non-tabletted one. An example thereof has been found in tablets of ergocaclciferol (2) (Fig. 7).

This model shows stability to be reduced by an increase of free enthalpy difference. The decomposition rate was accelerated by the compaction pressure and the activation caused by it. This transformation of mechanical into chemical energy (via the "structural energy") at the same time showed that the "activation theory of tablet

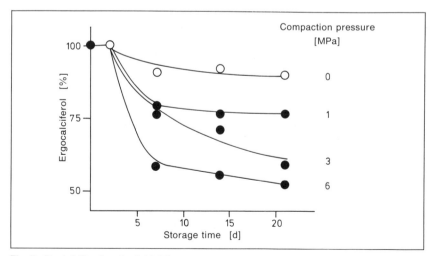

Fig. 7: Destabilization by tabletting

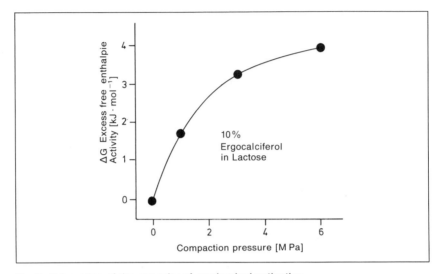

Fig. 8: Exhaustion of the capacity of mechanical activation

formation" had started from correct assumptions. Analogous energy transform-ations should be taken into consideration for all other mechanical operations. The induced agent degradation is a measure of the occurrence of activation, from which according to the EYRING equation follows the level of activation (3). With increasing mechanical loading it changes exponentially, until reaching a saturation (Fig. 8).

We have found that the excess free enthalpy in a lactose basis assumes a peak value of about 4 kJ/mol. It is noteworthy that trituration in a porcelain mortar yielded the same saturation value. At this limit the capacity of activation of the system or structure appears to be exhausted. This molecular-pharmaceutical finding explains some previously obscure decomposition processes. It also makes possible to determine a mechanical stress, such as compaction pressure, by a chemical method.

Besides, the example shows that our conceptions of the nature of solid matter should be changed basically. Solids generally are considered to be rigid, invariable and of poor reactivity. This is to be compared with what is known to use today, i.e. that a crystal is able to undergo growth and ageing, fatigue and recovery, that properties of it are inheritable, that it reacts to influences and adapts itself to its environment, shows a certain sensibility and is able to shout and even remember – that, as a matter of fact, it lives. And it changes its state of order spontaneously. It is the lattice defects that determine its temperament and "vitality". According to GEGUZIN each solid is at all times able to create itself the structure, which under the respective conditions is energetically most favourable to it. Consequently, it releases energy, if it has excess of it, changes its structure, if it dislikes it.

This adaptibility and "viability" is based upon the diffusion, the tendency of

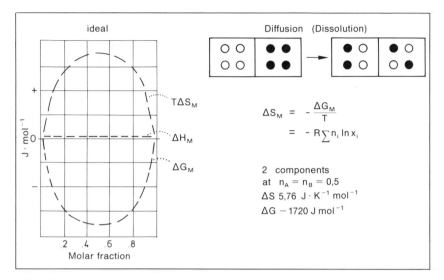

Fig. 9: Spontaneous uniform distribution of structural elements

substance components to distribute uniformly into one another with increasing entropy (entropy of mixing) (Fig. 9).

The entropy gain is dependent upon the mass ratio of the components and is highest with equality of concentration. In case of ideal conditions (without intermolecular interaction) and $\Delta H = 0$, it applies $\Delta S_M = \Delta G_M / T$.

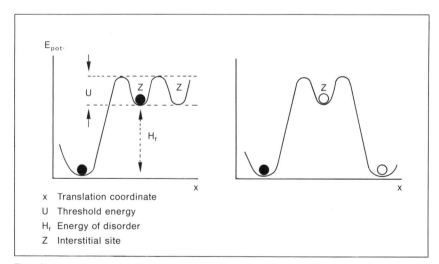

x   Translation coordinate
U   Threshold energy
H_f Energy of disorder
Z   Interstitial site

Fig. 10: Mechanism of diffusion

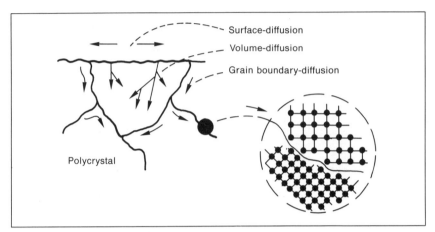

Fig. 11: Different types of diffusion

There is a close relationship between the molecular transport processes and the disorder, as interchange of molecules presupposes structural defects, while diffusion needs vacancy. The mobility of molecules results from their ability to exceed the sum of disorder energy and energy threshold and to move on by kangaroo jumps (Fig. 10).

Depending upon the molecules' migration path three kinds of diffusion can be distinguished: surface diffusion, volume diffusion, and grain boundary diffusion (Fig. 11).

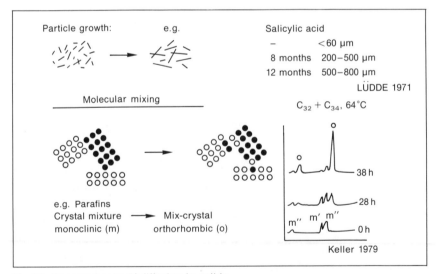

Fig. 12: Consequences of diffusion in solids

While at low and medium temperatures the grain boundary diffusion is predominant, the volume diffusion is predominant at high temperatures. The considerable differences between solids, liquids and gases are involved by the same cause as is the influence of temperature, i.e. by the varying portion of free spaces.

Of practical importance, as a consequence of self-diffusion, is particle growth, which can be remarkable in ground powders (4) (Fig. 12).

Small particles have a higher steam pressure (GIBBS-THOMSON equation) and a higher energy than large-sized ones; therefore the molecules in the course of their migration preferably leave the small particles to become attached to large-sized ones. This leads to the "OSTWALD ripening", i.e. the large particles grow at the expense of the small.

Another process underrated in the solid state is the molecular self-mixing of dry powders. Lattice elements which, forced by equipartition (entropy production), leave their crystals to penetrate into neighbouring ones cause mix-crystals to be formed spontaneously with the pertaining lattice imperfections (Fig. 12). In the case of paraffins, such spontaneous mixing was evident in the X-ray diffractogram already after few hours. Indicative of this was the fact that in mix-crystal formation the monoclinic modification simultaneously passes into an orthorhombic one (5). In metallurgy, the molecular transitions in metallic structures are referred to as diffusion alloying.

Solids' sintering uses the diffusion of vacancies (voids). Such change of the solids renders it possible to spontaneously reduce the free surface energy of the particles and at the same time anneal lattice defects under solidification and compaction. In pharmaceutics, the after-hardening of tablets represents a so-called dry sintering.

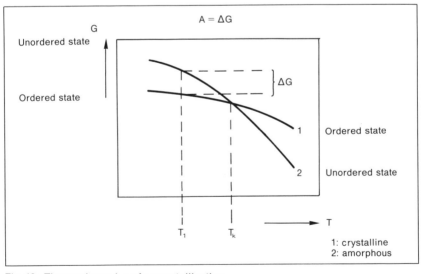

Fig. 13: Thermodynamics of recrystallization

Vacant sites have much higher migration rates than lattice elements. By way of example, in gold, the migration rate of vacancies at a temperature approaching the melting temperature is 10 km/h, whereas that of the atoms is as low as about 1 m/h, i.e. 10000 times lower. Starting from the above pattern of the diffusion mechanism the voids make 10 milliards of jumps per second. With rising temperature all crystals become more "vivid". In gold, e. g., the ratio of the unoccupied to the occupied lattice sites at room temperature amounts $1 : 10^{15}$, whereas at the melting point it is as low as $1 : 10^4$. The state of order changes exponentially. And since it is the disorder that forms diffusion channels and where runs the diffusion flow, also the properties of the materials while heated change exponentially.

To recapitulate, it should be noted that lattice defects are not only the "fuel", but also the transport paths for molecular masses and induce not only chemical reactions such as the ergocalciferol decomposition, but also physical processes such as grain growth, autogenous mix-crystal formation or spontaneous tablet solidification. However, in the simplest case, the solid matter frees itself from its metastable state by recrystallizing. The reason for this is again the free enthalpy difference (Fig. 13).

Below the melting point T_k, structurally defect, partially crystalline or even amorphous substances have a higher free enthalpy and hence pass spontaneously into the ordered state, whereas above the melting temperature, the free enthalpy of the crystals is predominant, so that during melting amorphous structures are formed. The recrystallization rate or rate of decay of the activated state is determined by the lifetime of the lattice defects. In a number of drugs the following course has been found (Fig. 14).

The phenomenon has proved strongly substance-involved. X-ray crystallography showed a rapid increase of crystallinity in digitoxin (6), whereas a structure-dependent quantity such as the angle of contact was used to determine the kinetics in ASS and yielded substantially higher values (7). The phase transition followed a first-order reaction. For indomethacin the ARRHENIUS diagramm was chosen in the plot, in order to demonstrate the temperature dependence of the change (8). The rates differ by orders of magnitude.

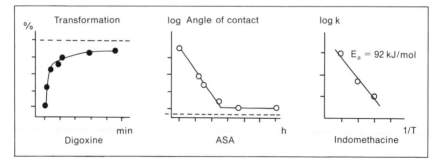

Fig. 14: Kinetics of recrystallization

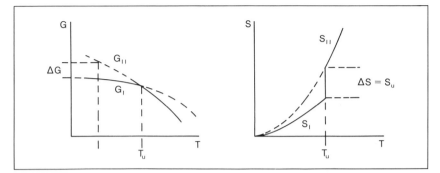

Fig. 15: Thermodynamics of polymorphous transformation

The interchanges of sites in the crystal lattice also include the polymorphic transformation. Again the events are directed by the differences of the free enthalpies and the entropy increases (Fig. 15).

Only at the transformation point T_u, where this difference is zero both crystal forms of an entity can stably coexist. The direction of change on both sides of the point is thermodynamically determined. Entropy plays an important role in the change of the free enthalpy. Frequently, the transformation temperature is relatively high, closely approaching the melting temperature, so that at room temperature transformation does not yet occur.

Different rules have been known, by which modification changes occur. One of them is the so-called density rule, which implies that of two modifications of a molecular crystal the one which has the higher density at r.t. is the more stable at absolute zero. Higher density means smaller molecular spacing and hence higher

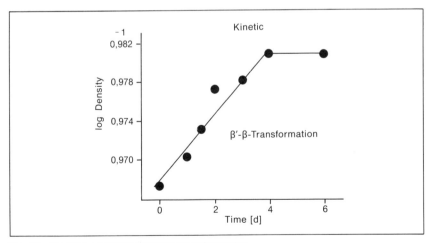

Fig. 16: Kinetics of polymorphous transformation

lattice energy and lower free enthalpy. Therefore we indirectly used the density rule to determine the kinetics of a polymorphic transformation. Selecting triglyceride suppository materials, the polymorphism of which had been subject to a variety of galenic investigations, we measured the change of density in dependence on time (9) (Fig. 16).

It has been evident from the findings that the transformation proceeds by a reaction of first order, and half-life is about 2200 hr, corresponding to 91 days. Much more rapid behaves the transformation of the α-form into the β-form, usually requiring but minutes. As to the β-β'-transformation other authors have found an activation energy of 410 kJ, from which follows a high temperature sensitivity of the process. Thus half-life at a temperature of 30 °C is as low as 48 hr, being reduced to 8 hr at a temperature of 34 °C (10). Since 1923, it has been known that the transformation is induced and enhanced not only by the thermal energy, but also by the mechanical energy. By grinding and pressing the lattices can be loosened and activated to such an extent that the structure "flops over". In the disordered regions of a polymorphic substance the crystallization process may realize another modification.

Still more easily do polymorphic transformations proceed in the presence of a liquid, which loosens the bonds differently. For instance, in suspensions the vehicle acts like that as a carrier. Frequently, the modification change is actually made possible by the suspending liquid. Part of the original solid matter is dissolved by the liquid and recrystallized into another crystal structure, with a lower energy barrier to be overcome than is the case in the dry state, solvation, however, not being required.

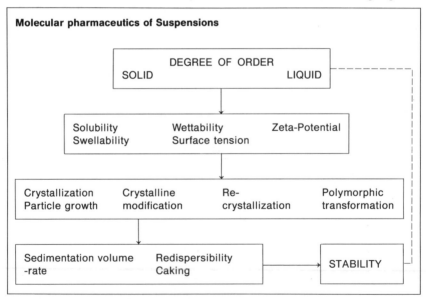

Fig. 17: Hierarchy of stability factors of suspensions

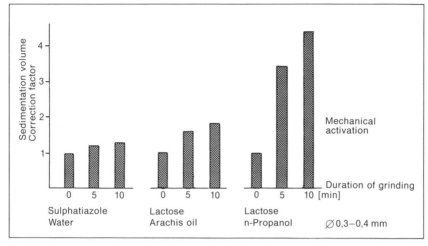

Fig. 18: Surface structure of particles and stability of suspensions

The mechanism results in that always the more slightly soluble form accumulates. So oxyclozamide while being rearranged at r.t. in aqueous suspension, does not show a phase change in the dry state even at temperatures ranging between −80 and +150°C (11). By the influence of the liquid on the structural dynamics in suspensions other processes such as the grain growth are also enhanced. The tendency to change always rises with the solubility (thermodynamic activity). In lyophilic systems lattice defects promote the processes, inter alia, by increasing the wettability and solubility of solids. For comparable reasons, the growth of specifically light particles is more rapid than that of specifically heavy ones.

Here should be pointed out that grain growth is possible not only in powders and suspensions, but also in tablets. In compacts it is induced due to stress differences, thus being called a "stress-induced grain growth". By reduction of the particle interface the system relaxes and stabilizes. Hence the particle size growth repeatedly demonstrated in tablets may be proportionally based on a secondary effect, too.

Returning to the complexity of the changes in suspensions, we state that again the state of order is a central quantity from which to derive the stability-governing factors (Fig. 17).

Studies undertaken during the last few years have provided evidence for the correlations including the importance of the electrokinetic potential. All effects finally lead to the stability criterion. The wettability example is to illustrate the matter (12) (Fig. 18).

The driving force of the process being directly correlated with the interfacial tension and the surface difference, the stability of a suspension will be the higher, the lower is the interfacial tension and the smaller is the particle-size difference. In all systems investigated interfacial (mechanical) activation caused the sedimentation volume to increase, while stability rose with the particles' wetting.

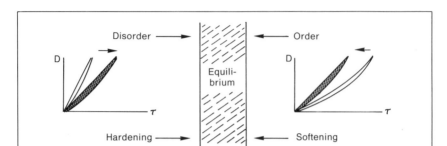

Fig. 19: Conflict of opposed forces in ointments

Solid-liquid systems of special kind are ointments, in which numerous phenomena remind of suspensions. However, the liquid phase in ointments not only plays a mediator role, but participates directly in structurization. This results in a novel structure type and a characteristic state of matter. The liquid phase is immobilized by the always lyophilic solid phase, both phases forming a unity.

Many ointments are subject to ageing; but the relevant data are controversal. Several authors found an increase of viscosity in the course of storage, whereas others found a decrease. Therefore the phenomenon was difficult to interpret. From the viewpoint of molecular pharmaceutics the following picture is offered (Fig. 19).

Ointments are characterized by the conflict of opposed forces, hence being always at strife structurally and thermodynamically. With regard to the solid-liquid balance crystallization and dissolution are competing. Both processes are not pure volume processes, but are essentially determined by interfacial effects. The volume term must be dominant, in order that the change of the free enthalpy assumes negative values; this tendency, however, being counteracted by the surface formation, which "curbs" the events. The difference between crystallization and dissolution consists in the total strain energy, which makes a positive or a negative contribution. A dislocation increasing the total strain energy would be promotive to dissolution and inhibitory to crystallization. In the case of real matters the free enthalpy difference of dissolution is always more strongly negative than it is in the case of ideal ones. A certain exception is formed by screw dislocations. They direct and facilitate the crystallization, enabling crystal growth at a rate 10^{1000} times higher than predetermined by theory.

Another rivalry consists between BERTHELOT's principle and the second law of thermodynamics. The former demands each system to strive for an energy minimum (i.e. removal of lattice defects, with only exothermic processes being spontaneous), whereas the latter is based on aiming at an entropy maximum, tantamount to an increase of defect and lattice imperfections.

Thus it was assumed that it depends on the respective molecular order of an ointment, in which direction its structure and properties are changed. With equal composition they always had to strive for the same dynamic balance. This meant that while a lack of disorder results in hardening (since lattice defects increase the strength), and increase of order results in softening. The conclusions were corroborated by the experiments (13) (Fig. 20).

When Polyethylene-ointments were fused and by shear crystallization adjusted to a different degree of order, they tended, during storage from either direction at the same state of equilibrium. This caused an after-hardening in relatively well-crystallized ointments and an after-softening in relatively poorly ordered ones.

Ointments are self-optimizing systems, self-acting to change their structure to arrive at the state, which is thermodynamically most favourable. It is their aim to realize a relatively high concentration of lattice defects in the solid phase, which corresponds to a criterion of existence of the high-liquid, spreadable, semisolid state. If such a "harmonization" between the phases fails to be achieved, there will be a partial separation such as in the case of syneresis or a complete separation as in the case of suspensions. The high plastic deformability would be unimaginable without the structural defects in the matrix. Therefore ointments are generally obtained via the melting phase, the melts being cooled down with stirring, in this way producing a high degree of disorder. With respect to the combination of different states of matter and different binding forces the constructive phase coexistence is based upon a structural and thermodynamic compromise between the extremes.

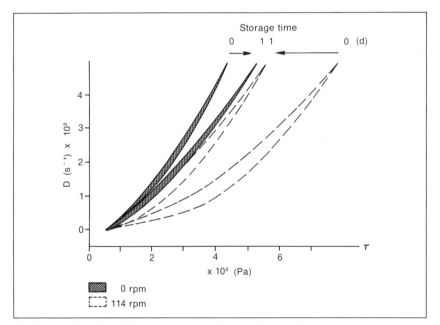

Fig. 20: Equilibration of forces and properties in ointments

3. Liquid dosage forms

The state of order of liquids is of similar galenic importance as that of solids. With suspensions and ointments, dosage forms have been treated above, whose properties are co-determined by the liquid structure. A lot of further systems contain a liquid component. Therefore molecular pharmaceutics has likewise to deal with these molecular foundations. The structural differences of the liquids vs. solids are by far smaller than is commonly assumed. Liquids are duly comprehended to be structurally defect solids. A relatively high degree of order is found especially in water as the most important solvent.

An influence on the water structure, properly speaking, is a change of structural dynamics and structural kinetics. The degree of order is correlated with the residence time of the water molecules. Increase of the molecules' rate of movement by temperature rise, e. g. will diminish the clusters, thus reducing the average extension of the short-range order zones around the individual water molecules (14) (Fig. 21).

This is to be compared with shifting the temperature towards the other side, which causes the spherical radii to increase; finally, at the freezing point, short-range order passes into long-range order, "short-range crystallinity" becoming "long-range crystallinity".

It is essential for pharmaceutics that zones of short-range order can be modified also by the presence of dissolved substances. In this concern, a distinction is to be made between compounds extending the zones or increasing the residence time of the molecules and such causing the opposite (15) (Fig. 22).

By comparison, I would like to suggest that the time between two interchange jumps in solids is 10^{-5}s and in water averages 10^{-11}s. Whereas the so-called structure-makers cause a positive hydration and dilate the hydrate envelope, structure-breakers cause a negative hydration, being even in a position to disintegrate the hydrate envelope completely. The structural effect is correlated with the potential

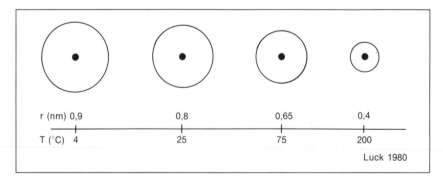

Fig. 21: Spherical radius of ordered zones as a measure of ordering in liquids

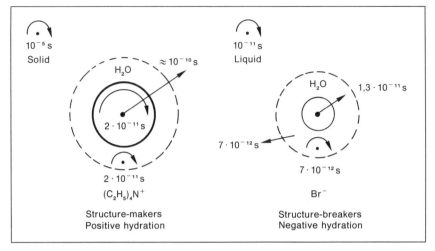

Fig. 22: Changing the extension of order by substances

barrier of hydration and the self-diffusion energy of water. The change of the quantities follows certain principles (Fig. 23).

In the case of (inorganic) electrolytes the self-diffusion energy decreases with increasing ionic radius of the added cations and likewise with diminishing ionic charge. This results in an increased motility and exchange rate of the water molecules. Whereas lithium and sodium ions still exert a positive influence, potassium and caesium ions act as structure breakers, leading to a negative hydration. The threshold is at a radius of 0,11 nm for monovalent cations. Multiple charged ions such as

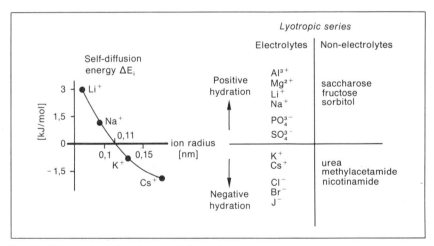

Fig. 23: Stepladders of order-modifying potencies

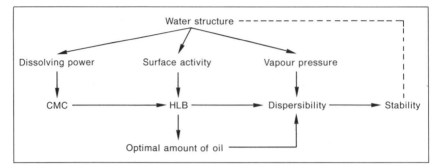

Fig. 24: Cooperation of stability factors in emulsions

aluminium and magnesium ions surpass the alkali ions. An analogous behaviour is shown by anions. Bringing the electrolytes into an order of sequence because of their influence on the water structure yields a correspondence with the so-called HOFMEISTER series or "lyotropic series of electrolytes" (see also the variation of the structural temperature according to LUCK) (14).

We have found even a "lyotropic series of non-electrolytes" to be existent (16). All non-ionics can be ranked in respect to their structure-increasing or structure-decreasing effectiveness, while ranking of all galenic agents or adjuvants is possible in dependence upon their influence on the water structure. In aqueous solutions a change in the liquid structure with its consequences should generally be taken into account.

The multiplicity of consequences include such processes as important as the evaporation of water, involved by changes in the surface tension and vapour pressure. We succeeded to demonstrate (17) that the evaporation rate is correlated with the water structure. Undesirable loss of moisture and intended drying may be delayed or enhanced by certain additives, there being a simple explanation for a varying behaviour of drug formulations.

Heterogeneous multiphase systems with an important role of the water component are represented by emulsions. As a matter of principle, dispersions are thermodynamically unstable, with different factors coming into question for the instability: all were unambiguously dependent on the water structure (18) (Fig. 24).

The sum of the effects was expressed in the influence of the water structure on the emulsions' tendency of separation. Relating to this, it was remarkable that the state of order of water had a much greater influence on the stability of W/O-emulsions than it had on the behaviour of O/W-emulsions. In addition, the separation was increased by structure makers in the case of W/O-emulsions, while in O/W-emulsions, it was reduced (19, 20) (Fig. 25).

Quite another type of molecular pharmaceutical structural effects relates to the function of water in the case of hydrophobic interactions. Since hydrophobic "bonds" determine, inter alia, the intramolecular state of order of the macro-molecules, the conformation of such molecules, in solution, is changed with the

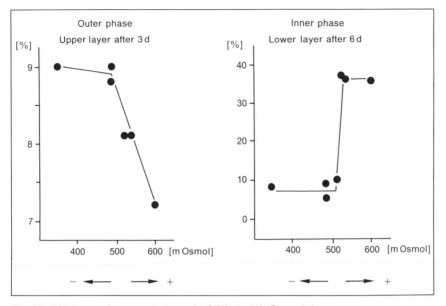

Fig. 25: Efficiency of water structure in O/W- and W/O-emulsions

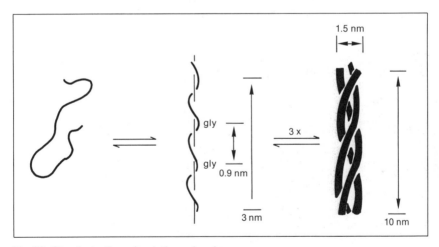

Fig. 26: Structurization of gelatin molecules

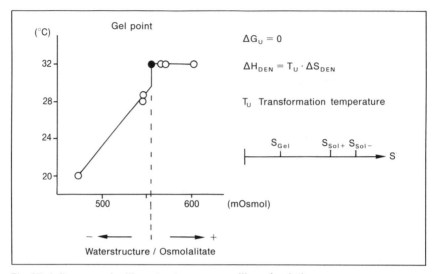

Fig. 27: Influences of milieu structure upon gelling of gelatin

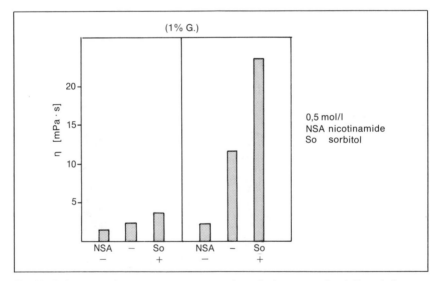

Fig. 28: Relevance of water structure upon viscosity increase of gelatin solutions

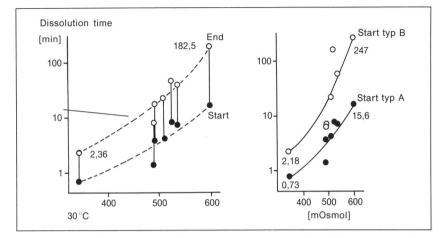

Fig. 29: Relevance of water structure upon disintegration of gelatin microcapsules

structure of the medium. Varying the water structure results, e. g. in a displacement of the helix-coil equilibrium of dissolved proteins. The significance of this correlation for pharmaceutics is illustrated through the use, as an example, of gelatin, the protein of the greatest galenic importance.

The structurization of gelatin proceeds in several steps (Fig. 26)

The disordered coils first of all are converted into single helices, which combine to form so-called triple helices, and ageing finally results in the development of three-dimensional networks from the helically coiled strands. The single helicalization proceeds within a relatively short time, 10^{-6} s, while the formation of the hydrophobic clusters takes as much as 10^{-3} s. This is to be compared with a half-life of about 10 s, which has been found for the involution of the native protein structure (ribonuclease). The gelation of gelatin presupposes that the molecules have a helical conformation. Solely in the helical state are the macromolecules in a position to build up higher structural units and induce a gelation. That is why the influence exerted on the first step decides on the course of all subsequent steps.

The tendency to gelate is reflected by the gel point of the protein. The dependence of this criterion on the water structure is relatively strong. In our experiments the gelling point of gelatin changed by 12 K (21) (Fig. 27).

Since at the transformation point the difference of the free enthalpies equals zero, the change of enthalpy at this point gets equal to the product obtained by multiplying the temperature by the change of entropy. Assuming that the gel has always the same entropy, the entropy difference in case of transformation from a structurally lessened sol is greater than it is from a structurally augmented sol. Consequently, the transformation point in the presence of structure breakers is lower than it is in pure water and lower, too, than it is with added structure makers. The transformation point, as it were, adapts itself to the entropy change. Naturally, there is a certain shift to be seen in the gelation enthalpy, too. For the helicalization, it is said to range generally from 2 to 34 KJ/mol. For the whole gelation, a value of 88 kJ/mol has been described.

As mentioned above, the single helix formation is prerequisite to all further structure changes. That is why the water structure controls the ageing of gelatin sols. The effects seen are noteworthy (22) (Fig. 28).

The ageing of a one per cent gelatin solution is about seven times more intense in the presence of the structure maker sorbitol than it is in the presence of the structure breaker nicotinamide (related to the factor of viscosity). By nicotinamide ageing is almost completely prevented.

Studying the reversed process, i. e. the dissolution of gelatin gels yields comparable results. So findings on microcapsules (using microexamination) revealed the disintegration times shown in Fig. 29 (23).

The picture of the great differences evident from the semilogarithmic plot is less striking. By modification of the water structure the beginning of the dissolution in one case varied from 2 to 247 min, while the end of the disintegration process extended over 8 hr. This great range over more than two orders of magnitude has several galenic consequences. Thus microcapsules serve to stabilize active substances such as vitamin A. This protection may get lost in the presence of nicotinamide, for example in polyvitamin preparations. Without the molecular pharmaceutical view, it would be impossible to trace the causality line of the unexpected high vitamin-A decomposition. Nowadays, it is wellknown that nicotinamide reduces the water structure, that in the structurally reduced medium the gelatin helices are despiralized, thus causing the gelatin gel point to drop and the microcapsules to disintegrate already at r. t., and that subsequently the readily oxidizable vitamin is released. If the molecular mechanism is known, the measures to stop the process are quite apparent.

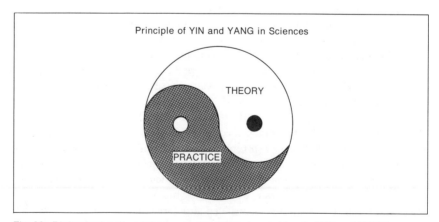

Fig. 30: Dialectical unity of theory and practice in analogy to YIN and YANG

4. Final remarks

The explanations show that the molecular theoretical view acts as an enormous magnifier: known effects can be seen through, new phenomena become visible, novel paths to a targetted influence on the processes are recognized. Hence, it appears to us that the YIN-YANG double image is transferable to the situation of applied sciences (Fig. 30).

Theory covers practice shelterlike, extending into it, being tantamount to it and essential for perfection of a discipline. Successful practice needs the base of theory. Yet, remember GOETHE, who once uttered thoughts, which could be expressed like this: A theory is like a scaffold, which is attached to a building and dismantled after its completion, being indispensable to the worker; only, he must not take the scaffold for the building.

References

(1) R. Hüttenrauch, Bedeutung des molekularen Ordnungszustands für Bildung und Verhalten der Arzneiformen, Symposium der Deutschen Akademie der Naturforscher Leopoldina, April 1984 in Halle/DDR; Nova Acta Leopoldina, in press
(2) R. Hüttenrauch und S. Fricke, Pharmazie *39*, 347 (1984)
(3) R. Hüttenrauch, S. Fricke und P. Zielke, Pharm. Res., 302 (1985)
(4) K.-H. Lüdde und U. Krähner, Pharmazie *26*, 507 (1971)
(5) G. Ungar und A. Keller, Colloid Polym. Sci. *257*, 90 (1979)
(6) D. B. Black und E. G. Lovering, J. Pharmacy Pharmacol. *30*, 380 (1978)
(7) R. Hüttenrauch, Pharmazie *39*, 272 (1984)
(8) H. Imaizumi, N. Nambu und T. Nagai, Chem. Pharm. Bull. (Tokyo) *28*, 2565 (1980)
(9) R. Hüttenrauch und U. Möller, Pharmazie *40*, 582 (1985)
(10) H. Yoshino, Y. Hagiwara, M. Kobayashi und M. Samejima, Chem. Pharm. Bull. (Tokyo) *32*, 1523 (1984)
(11) J. T. Pearson und G. Varney, J. Pharmacy Pharmacol., Suppl. *21*, 60 S (1969)
(12) R. Hüttenrauch und U. Möller, Pharmazie *38*, 198 (1983)
(13) R. Hüttenrauch, S. Fricke und V. Baumann, Pharmazie *37*, 25 (1982)
(14) W. Luck, Fortschr. chem. Forsch. *4*, 653 (1964)
(15) E. Wicke, Angew. Chem. *78*, 1 (1966)
(16) R. Hüttenrauch und S. Fricke, Pharmazie *37*, 720 (1982)
(17) R. Hüttenrauch und U. Möller, Pharmazie *37*, 301 (1982)
(18) R. Hüttenrauch und S. Fricke, Pharmazie *37*, 147, 300, 301, 720, 844 (1982); *38*, 129 (1983); *39*, 714 (1984)
(19) R. Hüttenrauch und U. Möller, Pharmazie *38*, 267 (1983)
(20) R. Hüttenrauch und P. Zielke, Pharmazie *38*, 492 (1983)
(21) R. Hüttenrauch und S. Fricke, Pharmazie *39*, 125 (1984)
(22) R. Hüttenrauch und S. Fricke, Naturwiss. *71*, 426 (1984); Pharmazie *39*, 501 (1984)
(23) R. Hüttenrauch und S. Fricke, Pharmazie, *41*, 515 (1986)

II. Physicochemical Criteria for semi-solid dosage forms

S.S. Davis, University of Nottingham, GB-Nottingham

1. Introduction

The purpose of this chapter is to consider the physicochemical changes that can occur is semi-solid dosage forms upon storage. Mollica et al (1) have provided a useful, but broad definition of pharmaceutical semi-solids; "It includes all dosage forms that are not true solutions or dry oral solids". This means ointments, creams, gels, suppositories, as well as more fluid systems such as emulsions and suspensions.

Instability in any pharmaceutical system can be attributed to one of three different mechanisms of degradation: – chemical, physical, microbiological.

The chemical stability of semi-solid dosage forms has been well described recently by Carstensen (2) from the standpoint of the formulated drug substance. In such cases it is often possible to use modifications of conventional stability equations in order to analyse stability data or to make predictions. However, when dealing with changes in physical stability one will be concerned with the drug substance contained within the formultion, and also, and perhaps more importantly, the properties of the vehicle itself.

Physical changes within the system will have three major consequences (3,4). (i) They may affect the appearance of the product (and also the odour and texture), (ii) they may affect dose uniformity, and (iii) they may affect the bioavailability of the product. These changes in turn may result in poor patient compliance or reduced or variable efficacy in treatment. Some relevant examples include phase separation in emulsion systems, the caking of a suspension at the bottom of a container, the sedimentation of drug particles in a semi-solid ointment leading to a non-uniform distribution of the active material through the mass, changes in crystal habit (polymorphism), change of solvation state, and particle growth (Ostwald ripening). The various types of semi-solid dosage form will be examined in turn to indicate where possible changes in physical properties can occur.

2. The various types of semi-solid forms

2.1 Suspensions

Changes in the properties of suspensions can be manifested in the following way: –
(i) Ostwald ripening (the change in the particle size of a system due to the higher

surface free energy of small particles as compared to large particles. As a result the particle size in the system gradually increases.) (5), (ii) Hydrate formation/solvate formation (6), (iii) Polymorphic changes (the conversion of one polymorphic form of a compound to a more stable but less soluble form) (7), (iv) Sedimentation of individual particles within the suspension (8), (v) the flocculation and aggregation of particles (3), (vi) the creation of a cake that would be difficult to redisperse (5).

2.2 Emulsions

The instability phenomena manifested by emulsions are similar in many respects to those demonstrated by suspensions (1), namely (i) Ostwald ripening (sometimes called molecular diffusion) that can lead to the formation of large emulsion droplets from smaller ones (9), (ii) Creaming of the emulsion system where a less dense layer of the oil phase rises to the top of the container (10). This layer can normally be redispersed, (iii) the flocculation and aggregation of an emulsion leading to a more rapid creaming and (iv) the possibility of coalescence between emulsion droplets leading to irreversible breakdown within the system and the separation of a free oil of the dispersed phase (3). With emulsion systems the disperse particles may be an active drug material in its own right or may be a vehicle containing a dissolved or dispersed drug. It should also be realised that a number of medicinal products are in the form of emulsions, for example products intended for parenteral nutrition (fat emulsions) or products used as red blood cell substitutes (11).

2.3 Suppositories

The commonly used suppository bases consist of complex mixtures of triglycerides. These triglyceride materials are able to undergo conversion from one polymorphic form to another more stable polymorphic form (7). Triglyceride species are able to exist in α, β, or β' polymorphic forms, therefore giving rise to a large number of possible transitions and as a consequence alteration in the melting point of a product upon storage. Suppositories containing disperse solids or liquids will also manifest the instability problems inherent in emulsion and suspension formulations (13).

2.4 Gels

Gel systems can be produced from natural and synthetic materials such as polymers. Changes can take place in the structure of gels leading to alteration in rheological properties (14). This may in turn affect the stability of a suspended material, eg resulting in coalescence or caking phenomena.

2.5 Ointments and creams

These categories of pharmaceutical product are normally complex versions of suspensions, emulsions and gels. Thus, one or more of the following stability problems can take place (3), (i) Ostwald ripening, (ii) polymorphic changes, (iii) sedimentation, (iv) rheological changes, (v) bleeding (the separation of continuous phase), (vi) evaporation of constituents.

3. Evaluation of physicochemical properties

From what has been discussed so far it can be seen that pharmaceutical semi-solids can undergo a number of physicochemical changes. It is therefore not surprising to find that a large number of different techniques will be needed in order to evaluate changes in relevant parameters. The list will include: –

– particle size
– polymorphic-hydration-solvation states
– sedimentation-creaming
– caking-coalescence
– consistency
– drug release.

Under each of these headings it is possible to suggest methods and equipment that may prove to be suitable for the purpose required. However, it should be stressed that the technique employed should provide objective data on the observed changes without being over-complicated. In many instances it is possible to undertake highly sophisticated analyses of physicochemical changes, but all that may be required for product registration and for quality control purposes, is a much simpler investigation.

Particle size determinations include the classical microscope methods, but also more complex techniques such as the Coulter Counter, photon correlation spectroscopy (for very small particles) and other techniques that can provide relative data on size and size distribution; for example diffuse reflectance (15) and the measurement of ultrasound (16). Proper attention to the relevance and sophistication of the chosen method can be illustrated by recent studies on the stability of fat emulsions intended for parenteral nutrition (17). The test emulsions were subjected to accelerated testing in the form of a standardised shaking test and particle size analysis was conducted by three methods: – (i) Microscopic observation for large particles, (ii) Coulter Counter for medium-sized particles and (iii) Photon correlation spectroscopy for small particles.

In a typical bottle of 1 litre of fat emulsion, there will be about 10^{15} particles. The method adopted should therefore be relevant to the final use of the system and with regard to the probable consequences of changes in the stability parameter. When the emulsion was examined by photon correlation spectroscopy (a method that looks at the very small particles) it would appear that the particle size had decreased slightly (Figure 1). However, using the Coulter Counter, where particles above about 1 micron in size were examined, it was clear, that the system was far from stable.

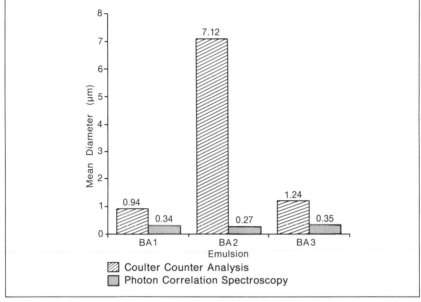

Fig. 1: The particle size analysis of fat emulsions subjected to accelerated testing (shaking test).

Indeed, visual and microscopic examination demonstrated the presence of free oil on the surface of the emulsion system! These large droplets of free oil would obviously have an important bearing on toxicity but an insignificant effect on the total number of droplets and the measured mean *number* diameter obtained by photon correlation spectroscopy.

3.1 Crystalline properties

Changes in crystal structure due to polymorphism, hydration or solvation can be measured using X-ray methods or by differential thermal analysis and differential scanning calorimetry (6, 7). Figure 2 shows changes in X-ray diffraction patterns for prednisolone as it changes from an anhydrous form to a hydrate in an oil in water emulsion formulation. Such polymorphic changes may have a dramatic effect upon the release properties of the drug from an ointment (Figure 3). The technique of differential thermal analysis (DTA) has been used to follow the increase in the melting point of fatty suppository bases on storage. This change can be closely associated with the conversion of the α, and β' polymorphs of the constituent bases to the more stable β polymorph (12).

3.2 Sedimentation and creaming

The instability within a disperse system can be defined by Stokes' equations (or modifications thereof) (5) and measured by visual examination, ultrasound, conductivity etc. With suspensions the properties of a suspension can be determined by the measurement of a sedimentation volume (8). This parameter provides information as to the flocculated or unflocculated nature of the suspension.

3.3 Consistency

The term consistency is used to provide a general and non-specific term for physical quantities that are better represented in terms of the absolute parameters viscosity and elasticity (18). While it is easy to talk about the "viscosity" of a simple liquid, more complicated pharmaceutical materials like semi-solids are viscoelastic and these systems are notoriously difficult to characterise using simple tests. Correct rheological characterisation can be carried out using sophisticated tests (eg so-called creep and oscillatory experiments) but some information can be provided by less complex continuous shear determinations. The applicability of the test very much depends

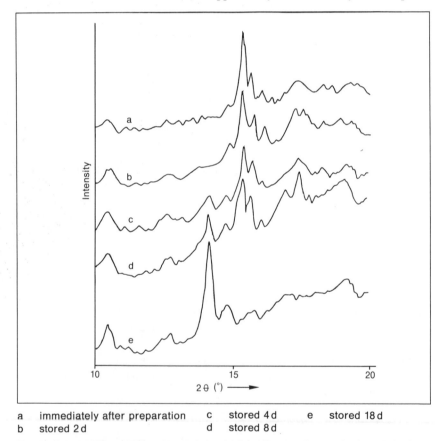

a   immediately after preparation   c   stored 4 d   e   stored 18 d
b   stored 2 d   d   stored 8 d

Fig. 2: Change of X-ray diffraction patterns for prednisolone from anhydrous to hydrate form in an o/w type ointment (from Ref. 6).

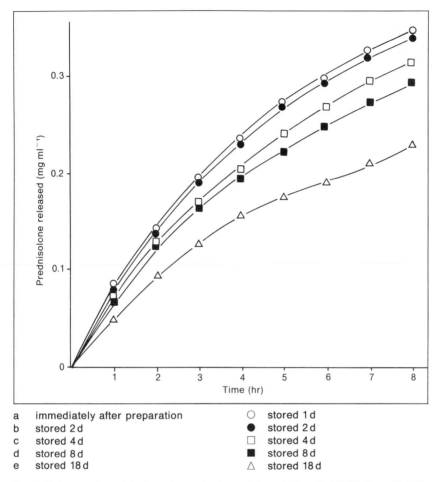

a	immediately after preparation	○	stored 1 d
b	stored 2 d	●	stored 2 d
c	stored 4 d	□	stored 4 d
d	stored 8 d	■	stored 8 d
e	stored 18 d	△	stored 18 d

Fig. 3: Release of prednisolone from o/w type ointment stored at 37 °C (from Ref. 6).

upon the structure of the system being examined and its elastic nature. Unfortunately, the literature contains continuous shear studies on ointments which present data that are almost totally worthless (18). The major problem is the inappropriateness of the test, a solid has been tested as if it were a liquid. In some viscometers it is apparent that the test sample has been ejected from the measuring surfaces of the instrument (19). But if unnoticed these experimental artefacts can be highly misleading, particularly when one examines changes taking place under storage. For example, if a system becomes less elastic (ie that is it has less structure) less of the material is expelled from the apparatus and more of the material will remain within the instrument to be measured during the experimental procedure. Thus it will appear that the material has gained consistency upon storage! The change in creep compliance of a water-in-oil emulsion after different ageing times is shown in Figure 4 (20). The compliance increases with storage time (that is the material is becoming more fluid and is losing structure). Such creep curves can be analysed in terms of a mechanical model from which fundamental rheological parameters can be calculated. However, each curve will require as many as six different parameters to describe the various elements within the rheological model (20). A more appropriate parameter for stability testing and data reporting might be the measured compliance at a selected time (21).

Changes in viscoelastic properties may be more sensitive than measurements made using simple continuous shear measurements (22). Data presented by Eccleston (21) illustrate this point well. She measured some cosmetic creams and studied the apparent viscosity as determined by continuous shear, as well as the viscoelastic parameters, dynamic viscosity and elasticity obtained by oscillatory experiments. The experimental measurements of viscoelasticity were able to provide far better resolution of the properties of the different formulations than the corresponding

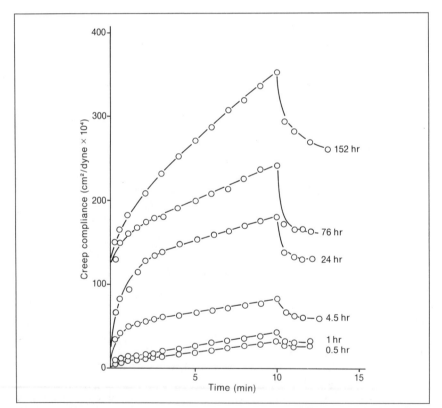

Fig. 4: Creep compliance of 50% (w/w) w/o emulsions after different ageing times (from Ref. 20).

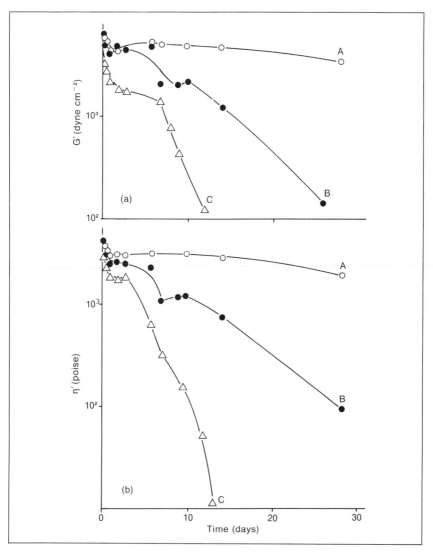

A   cetostearyl alcohol
B   cetyl alcohol
C   stearyl alcohol

Fig. 5: Variation of (a) storage modulus (G') and (b) dynamic viscosity (η') at fixed frequency (0.08 Hz) with storage time (from Ref. 21).

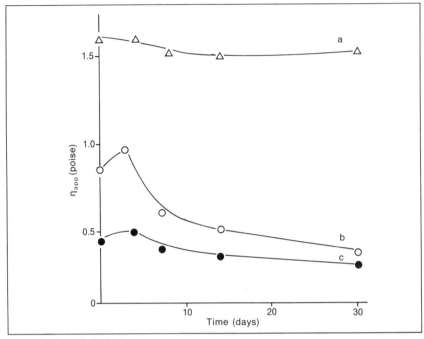

a   cetostearyl alcohol
b   cetyl alcohol
c)   stearyl alcohol

Fig. 6: Variation of apparent viscosity from continuous shear experiment (1671 sec^{-1}) with storage time (from Ref. 21).

continuous shear determinations (Figures 5, 6). Other empirical tests that have been helpful for the evaluation of consistency have been penetrometers and techniques to follow the extrusion of a product through an orifice or the spreading of the product on the skin (1, 4, 23).

Changes is consistency that can lead to an altered consumer evaluation, can be very difficult to measure in quantitative terms (20). Some success has been achieved in the field of cosmetics and the analysis of texture. However, parameters such a smoothness, stiffness, grittiness, greasiness and tackiness may be quite well understood in subjective terms but are not simple to evaluate objectively (3).

Creams containing glyceryl monostearate soap and water have been investigated using X-ray and thermal analytical methods (24). Upon cooling from the fused state the glyceryl monostearate molecule can assume the metastable α form which will differ in both structure and mechanical behaviour from the stable β forms. Transition from α to the β form then occurs during storage. These changes can be detected by determining the viscoelastic properties of the creams over an extended period of time. Such changes in the consistency of semi-solids, ointments and creams are not unusual

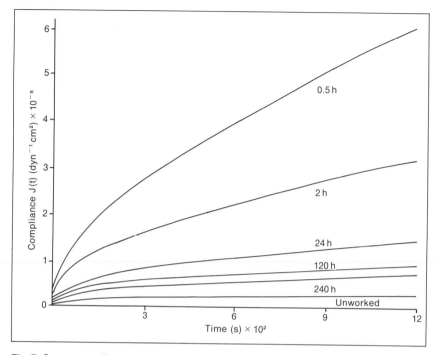

Fig. 7: Creep compliance curves indicating changes in viscoelastic behaviour of white soft paraffin BP after working (from Ref. 25).

(22). Even in the food industry, hardening of materials is a well recognised phenomenon that has been related to crystal growth (20). Figure 7 shows how the creep copliance properties of white soft paraffin BP are changed by working and then how the material can recover over a period of 10 days after working (25).

Viscoelastic networks within gel systems made from long chain alcohols and surfactants have been well described by Barry and Eccleston (21, 22). Such changes would indicate that rheological data obtained on freshly prepared semi-solids may not be correct (4).

One major disadvantage of the repeated rheological evaluation of stored systems is that the sample has to be removed from its container in order to fill a viscometer. This can disturb the structure that one wishes to measure! The penetrometer has an advantage in that it does not necessarily disturb the sample greatly. However, with most penetrometer geometries it is not possible to analyse the data in an objective way or to calculate viscoelastic parameters. An exception is the use of a spherical indenter that can be placed on a freshly prepared surface of a semi-solid and the movement of the indenter into the material can followed with some suitable optical or electrical arrangement (18, 26).

4. Accelerated tests

Those familiar with the testing of the chemical stability of pharmaceuticals will be aware of the utility of accelerated tests. These usually involve elevated temperature and in some cases high humidity. The results obtained can then be employed in predicitve assessments, often through the use of the simple Arrhenius equation. Accelerated tests can also be undertaken to examine changes in physical stability but often the results are of questionable value and exact predictive relationships are lacking (5, 27). Some of the accelerated methods that have been proposed include (i) elevated temperature, (ii) temperature cycling (to include freeze-thaw cycles), (iii) centrifugation and (iv) shaking tests.

The minimum temperature for temperature cycling is a matter of debate (5). For many products 5° is used as the lowest temperature but there are workers who prefer to get down to $-5\,°C$. Certainly with some systems (eg emulsions and suspensions) this lower temperature may cause irreversible changes and phase separation (28). These high stress conditions may be useful in ranking formulations on a comparative basis but they are not usually predictive of performance under conditions of normal storage. The reason for this is clear. Unlike chemical stability there are no exact relationships or equations that can be used for predictive purposes. In addition, the accelerated tests for physical stability may introduce conditions that do not operate under normal storage. For example, the centrifugation of emulsions has been found by many authors to be a useful parameter for assessing stability (10, 29–31), but this test can be criticised on the grounds that the centrifugal stresses often employed can

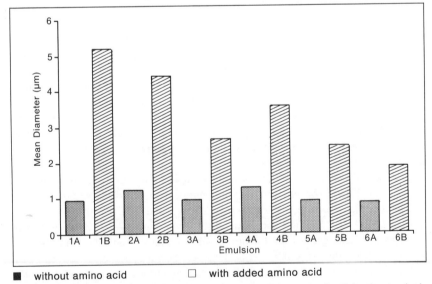

■ without amino acid   ☐ with added amino acid

Fig. 8: The stability of fat emulsions after one freeze thaw cycle. Particle size analysis conducted using a Coulter Counter (from Ref. 32).

cause deformations and changes in the structure of emulsions that do not occur under normal gravitational conditions. The aqueous phase can be separated from the emulsion and the oil globules are in close contact with each other forming distorted polyhedral shapes. Correlation of the shelf life stability with centrifugal stability requires a much deeper understanding of the mechanisms involved in centrifugal demulsification than is presently available (30).

As a general rule it can be stated that systems that withstand accelerated stress conditions should be stable under normal storage conditions. However the corollary is not necessarily true, namely that a system that is unstable under accelerated tests may not necessarily be unstable under normal storage. In our own studies we have found that the freeze-thaw cycle is a useful way of distinguishing stable fat emulsions from less stable systems in respect to long term stability and the effect of added electrolytes.

The data shown in Figure 8 are from six emulsion formulations containing slightly different proportions of fat, electrolyte, carbohydrate in the presence and absence of added amino acid. The systems were subjected to one freeze-thaw cycle and particle size analysis was conducted using the Coulter Counter. The dramatic destabilizing effect of the amino acid is well predicted (32).

5. Predictive methods

The sedimentation of a suspension or the creaming of an emulsion can be estimated by the application of Stokes' law, provided that the important parameters in the Stokes' equation can be measured or estimated, namely the mean particle size, the viscosity or the medium and the densities of the suspended material and the continuous phase (5). Also, it should be remembered that the equation is only valid for dilute systems. Once significant particle-particle interactions take place the original equation needs to be modified as described within the pharmaceutical and chemical engineering literature.

The process of Ostwald ripening has been discussed in mathematical terms by a number of authors including the original work conducted by Lord Kelvin (9). Some estimate of the importance of Ostwald ripening can be obtained if the solubility of the suspended material in the continuous phase of the system can be measured or calculated, as well as some knowledge of the particle size of the product being available. The process of Ostwald ripening can be hindered and almost eliminated by the use of suitable excipients that will provide an interfacial barrier to diffusion (7).

As a general rule it is very difficult to predict the stability of semi-solid materials. For example ointments and creams may undergo the phenomenon of bleeding and this irreversible change cannot be predicted in any meaningful way (3).

For the case of disperse systems it is possible to undertake calculations on stability using the so-called DLVO theory of colloid stability, provided some basic information is known; mean particle size, surface charge (zeta potential) and the presence (if any) of an adsorbed polymer layer and its thickness. Using this theory it is possible to construct potential energy-distance graphs and have some idea about the effect of an added components such as electrolytes (5, 33).

Other predictive methods for emulsion systems are based upon experimental determinations (29) and include the freeze-thaw test mentioned above, coalescence measurements (31, 34), centrifugation (10) and the measurement of phase inversion temperatures (35, 36). Tingstad (31) suggested that studies on the coalescence of oil droplets at the plane oil-water interface conducted using a coalescence cell arrangement, could provide information on the stability of emulsions made on a commercial scale. Some authors have found this method to be a useful approach, especially if the emulsifying agents are of natural origin and provide a thick interfacial layer at the oil-water interface (34). Unfortunately this predictive method has not been very successful for emulsions produced using emulsifying agents of low molecular weight (37). Clearly the forces operating between a plane oil-water interface and an oil droplet of millimetre dimensions are not the same as those operating between spherical particles of a micron size and less in emulsions.

Properly conducted centrifugation experiments can be used for predicting the stability of emulsion systems (10). In one such method phase separation is measured

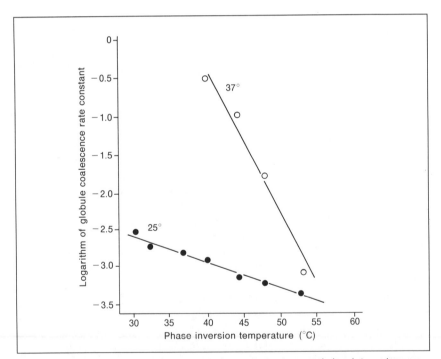

Fig. 9: Correlation between phase inversion temperature and droplet coalescence (from Ref. 35).

over a range of centrifugal speeds and a stability parameter, the coalescence pressure, can be calculated (38).

One method that holds promise for predicting the stability of emulsions prepared using non-ionic surfactants is based upon good correlations that exist between coalescence rates (and hence stability) and the phase inversion temperature (35, 36). The phase inversion temperature is the temperature where an oil-in-water emulsion changes into the reverse system, a water-in-oil emulsion. This change is related to the solubility of the emulsifier in water. Publications by Sherman (36), Enever (35) and Frankel and Garti (39) have indicated good log-linear relationships can be obtained between emulsion stability and phase inversion temperatures (Figure 9).

Attempts have been used to use rheological data to predict the storage stability of pharmaceutical suspensions (40). The method is apparently based upon the fact that flocculated suspensions will demonstrate a departure from Newtonian behaviour and that flocculation *per se* renders the system liable to caking and poor redispersibility. However, this may not be a generally applicable rule. Certainly our own studies on emulsions have shown that poor stability in terms of rapid flocculation and rapid creaming do not necessarily undergo coalescence. Emulsion systems stabilised by simple soaps were highly aggregated and at a 10% disperse phase volume underwent complete creaming within about 1–2 hours (disperse phase at the top of the container and a clear disperse phase underneath). However, no coalescence occurred since there was no noticeable change in mean particle diameter over a period of three years (as determined by Coulter Counter measurements) (41).

Some reports have suggested that there are possible correlations between zeta potential changes and accelerated ageing tests (42). In our view, changes in zeta potential in complex disperse systems are simply a manifestation of alterations in interfacial properties and it is doubtful whether they could be used for predictive purposes unless zeta potential values were employed in calculations of repulsive energy barriers using the DLVO theory as discussed earlier.

6. Protocols for the evaluation of physical stability

Because of the diversity of the different systems that come under the heading of pharmaceutical semi-solids, it is not possible to lay down detailed protocols for stability testing. However, the following should be borne in mind when designing future tests.

(i)   Store at selected temperatures and humidity conditions (the normal procedure for stability investigations)
(ii) Consider the utility of accelerated tests in the form of centrifugation or temperature cycling
(iii) Conduct shipping tests.

The last is appropriate since pharmaceutical suspensions, emulsions and semi-solids are complex systems and external physical influences like vibration can take place under shipping and transportation and can provide a source of possible major stress (4). In our own studies we use a shaking test (2–3 Hertz) to render normally stable fat emulsions (such as Intralipid) unstable over a period of a few hours. While we employ this method for accelerated stability testing, pharmaceutical systems may well be subjected to this type of mechanical stress during shipping and transport.

7. Stability Limits and conclusions

When discussing chemical instability it is normal pratice to consider a two-year shelf life and a stability limit of not more than a 10% change in the active principle. However, for changes in physical properties it is not always possible to set rigorous limits and only guidelines can be given. Unacceptable changes in drug release, that can be related to particle growth or change in crystal form, can be defined with appropriate limits. Changes in consistency and visual appearance are a different matter.

The first important matter to consider is the nature of the physical change taking place and its possible consequence. For example, a change in the particle size of a suspended drug may give rise to changes in dissolution and drug release which could affect the bioavailability of the compound. Polymorphic changes may similarly alter the solubility of the compound and its subsequent dissolution and release characteristics. Such alterations in the availability of the compound from the delivery system could be measured by conventional *in vitro* dissolution tests and a limit then set comparing the stored sytem with the original material.

Rheological changes in the vehicle may lead to unacceptable changes in terms of sedimentation or creaming. There are also implications on chemical stability because the diffusion coefficient of a drug is inversely proportional to the viscosity and it follows that the more viscous the preparation the more stable it will be from a chemical standpoint (2). Rheological changes that may alter consumer acceptance and preference are much more difficult to quantify or indeed to set limits.

Physical changes that can alter the performance of a product in the hands of the patient may allow reasonably broad limits. For example, a suspension that is undergoing an ageing process may be more difficult to resuspend. However, it the product can still be suspended in an acceptable period of time, the physical change should not lead to any serious effect on the efficacy of the product. But, if irreversible processes take place, such as caking or phase separation, this could have a dramatic effect upon patient acceptability as well as dose uniformity.

In some cases, changes in the physical properties of a system may well have implications not just for drug release but also for the toxicity of the product. A clear situation exists for an emulsion intended for intravenous administration, where coalescence and the separation of free oil would lead to dramatic toxic manifestations. An excessive increase in the particle size of an intravenous emulsion should not be tolerated but it is almost impossible to set a realistic limit. As shown previously the results on the physical stability of such systems can be influenced by the nature of the test being carried out. Particle size data can be biased to the lower end of the distribution curve if there were large numbers of small particles. Consequently the presence of larger particles could be overlooked when these would be far more relevant in terms of toxicity. The literature on intravenous fat emulsions suggests that particles greater than about 5 microns can cause problems in terms of entrappment in the capillary beds of the lung and the creation of lung emboli. Therefore it is not unreasonable in a pharmacopoeial monograph to set a limit that "the diameter of globules of the disperse phase of emulsions should not exceed 5 micron". Indeed this is the statement within the current European Pharmacopoeia and other national pharmacopoeias. But these pharmacopoeias give no information as to how determinations will be carried out or consider the impossibility of sampling every particle in a bottle of intravenous fat emulsion! One notes with satisfaction that in the revised version of the European Pharmacopoeia monograph on parenteral infusions, it states that "emulsions for intravenous infusion should not show any evidence of phase separation. The diameter of globules of the disperse phase of emulsions for intravenous infusion must be verified with regard to the use of the preparation". It has been realised that the 5 micron limit originally put forward, although admirable in concept, is an impossible to apply. Broad statements that leave the onus on the manufacturer could constitute acceptable available limits. Thus, we could state that the physicochemical changes that can occur within a semi-solid preparation upon storage or after processing (43) or other external influence, should not be such that they can alter the therapeutic efficacy of the product. This all encompassing requirement then places responsibility on the manufacturer to ensure that any changes in physical stability do not have a consequence for the proper use of the product by the patient and the release of the drug material from the dosage form. The guidelines for registration of new products with the Committee on Safety of Medicines in the United Kingdom apparently follow this line. They indicate that "evidence is required to demonstrate that the proposed formulation is stable for the purposes intended. It should meet the finished product specification throughout its self life".

References

(1) Mollica, J.A., Ahuja, S. and Cohen, J., J. Pharm. Sci. *67*, 443 (1978).
(2) Carstensen, J.T., Drug Devel. Ind. Pharm. *10*, 1277 (1984).
(3) Flynn, G.L., in G.F. Banker and C.T. Rhodes (Eds.), Modern Pharmaceutics, Marcel Dekker, New York, 263, 1979.
(4) Lintner, C.J., in A. Osol (ed.), Remington's Pharmaceutical Sciences, 15th edn., Mack, Philadelphia, 1425, 1975.

(5) Rhodes, C.T., in G.F. Banker and C.T. Rhodes (Eds.), Modern Pharmaceutics, Marcel Dekker, New York, 329, 1979.

(6) Kaiho, F., Goto, Y. and Kato, Y., Chem. Pharm. Bull. *28*, 2240 (1980).

(7) Haleblian, J. and McCrone, W., J. Pharm. Sci. *58*, 911 (1969).

(8) Law, S.L. and Kayes, J.B., Int. J. Pharmaceut. *15*, 251 (1983).

(9) Davis, S.S., Round, H.P. and Purewal, T.S., J. Colloid Interface Sci. *80*, 508 (1981).

(10) Garrett, E.R., J. Pharm. Sci. *54*, 1557 (1965).

(11) Davis, S.S., Hadgraft, J. and Palin, K.J. in P. Becher, Encyclopedia of Emulsion Technology, Vol. II, Marcel Dekker, New York, 159, 1985.

(12) Liversidge, G., Grant, D.J.W. and Padfield, J.M., Int. J. Pharmaceut. *7*, 211 (1981).

(13) Noro, S., Komatsu, Y. and Uesugi, T., Chem. Pharm. Bull. *30*, 2906 (1982).

(14) Barry, B.W. and Meyer, M.C., Int. J. Pharmaceut. *2*, 1 (1979).

(15) Akers, M.J. and Lach, J.L., J. Pharm. Sci. *65*, 216 (1976).

(16) Rassing, J. and Attwood, D., Int. J. Pharm. *13*, 47 (1983).

(17) Davis, S.S. and Galloway, M., To be published.

(18) Davis, S.S., In H. Asche, D. Essig and P.C. Schmidt (Eds.), Technologie von Salben, Suspensionen und Emulsionen, Wissenschaftliche Verlagsgesellschaft, Stuttgart, 160 (1984).

(19) Davis, S.S., Shotton, E. and Warburton, B., J. Pharm. Pharmacol. *20*, 1575 (1968).

(20) Sherman, P., Industrial Rheology, Academic Press, London, 1970.

(21) Eccleston, G.M., J. Colloid Interface Sci. *57*, 66 (1976).

(22) Barry, B.W., Advan. Pharm. Sci. *4*, 1 (1974).

(23) Ward, J.B., Kinney, J.F. and Saad, H.Y., J. Soc. Cosmet. Chem. *25*, 437 (1974).

(24) Klokkers, K. and Fuhrer, C., Acta Pharm. Technol. *31*, 151 (1985).

(25) Barry, B.W. and Grace, A.J., J. Pharm. Sci. *60*, 1198 (1971).

(26) Davis, S.S., Pharm. Acta Helv. *49*, 161 (1974).

(27) Rhodes, C.T., Drug Devel. Ind. Pharm. *5*, 573 (1979).

(28) Nakamura, A. and Okada, R., Colloid Polym. Sci. *254*, 718 (1976).

(29) Ondracek, J., Boller, F.H., Zullinger, H.W. and Niederer, R.R., Acta Pharm. Technol. *31*, 42 (1985).

(30) Hahn, A.U. and Mittal, K.L., Colloid Polym. Sci. *257*, 959 (1979).

(31) Tingstad, J.E., J. Pharm. Sci. *53*, 995 (1964).

(32) Davis, S.S., Galloway, M., Burnham, W.R. and Stevens, L., Clinical Nutrition *5*, 21 (1986).

(33) Davis, S.S., in I.D.A. Johnson (Ed.), Advances in Clinical Nutrition, MTP Press, Lancaster, 213, 1983.

(34) Davis, S.S. and Smith, A., Colloid Polym. Sci. *254*, 82 (1976).

(35) Enever, R.P., J. Pharm. Sci. *65*, 517 (1976).

(36) Parkinson, C.J. and Sherman, P., Colloid Polym. Sci. *255*, 172 (1977).

(37) Hansrani, P.K., PhD Thesis, Nottingham University, 1980.

(38) Buscall, R., Davis, S.S. and Potts, D.C., Colloid Polym. Sci. *257*, 636 (1979).

(39) Frenkel, M. and Garti, N., Thermochimica Acta *42*, 265 (1980).

(40) Caramella, C., Colombo, P., Conte, U. and LaManna, A., Il Farmaco (Ed. Pract.), *29*, 318 (1974).

(41) Davis, S.S. and Shotton, E., J. Pharm. Pharmacol. *20*, 439 (1968).

(42) Rambhau, D., Phadke, D.S. and Dorle, A.K., J. Soc. Cosmet. Chem. *28*, 183 (1977).

(43) Davis, S.S., Khanderia, M.S., Adams, I., Colley, I.R., Cammack, J. and Sanford, T., J. Texture Studies *8*, 61 (1977).

III. Physico-chemical criteria for the stability and stability forecast of solid dosage forms

M. Baltezor, Marion Laboratories Kansas City, Missouri

1. Introduction

The evaluation of the physico-chemical stability of a given solid dosage form requires first of all an understanding of the physical and chemical properties of the drug substance. Factors which are extremely critical to consider are the decomposition pathways, solubility, pKa, melting point, presence or absence of polymorphic crystal forms, and hydroscopic nature of the drug. Further, the combined effects of heat and moisture as well as light must be evaluated.

Once a drug substance is characterized in its pure form, the compatibility of the drug with the various excipients must also be considered. In order to successfully manufacture a drug product which can deliver a drug in a desired fashion, it becomes necessary to combine the pure drug substance with various fillers, binders, lubricants, disintegrants or retardation polymers. Additionally, the decomposition products of the drug must be considered as to their effect on the drug to insure that self-catalyzed decomposition does not occur.

The goal of the remainder of this paper will be to consider various physical tests which are commonly conducted on solid dosage forms and to attempt to derive a correlation between the results of these tests and the ultimate long term stability of the dosage form. Those physical tests which will be discussed will be sensory properties, hardness, moisture, disintegration time and rate of dissolution.

The definition of the actual testing conditions and environmental stresses can differ greatly between countries. From a purely scientific view, an investigator is free to design stress storage conditions which can be focused at the weak points of the dosage form. The severity of these stress conditions is often varied to yield results in a convenient time period. From a practical view, certain definitions of testing conditions need to be established. This allows different formulations and different products to be evaluated for their relative sensitivity toward environmental stresses. Also, on an industrial scale, it permits large storage chambers to be maintained for multiple product studies. For international firms with multicenter dosage form development activities, the consistency of storage conditions is imperative to allow meaningful comparisons of stability data between investigators at different sites.

Within the Sandoz organization, storage conditions have evolved over the years to both allow a scientifically meaningful challenge of the stability weak points of a drug product and to fit as well as possible the regulatory requirements imposed by various countries. Recently, our stability storage conditions were reviewed and set at − 25 °C, 5 °C, 25 °C with 50% R.H., 30 °C with 65% R.H., 30 °C with 75% R.H., 40 °C with less than 40% R.H. and 50 °C with less than 20% R.H. With these storage conditions plus some speciality storage conditions and tests such as high intensity light exposure, we have been able to both evaluate our formulations technically and to satisfy the needs of most regulatory requirements.

2. Sensory properties

The most apparent instability to a patient or pharmacist are changes in physical appearance (color, odor, taste, etc.). These traits also remain one of the most subjective in terms of monitoring them and translating changes into a numeric system.

Numerous researchers have investigated methods of monitoring changes in color. One source of discoloration is caused by darkening of tablets. This has emerged as an even larger problem with the increase in white tablets due to regulatory problems with various synthetic dyes. It has been demonstrated that darkening of a tablet follows zero or first oder kinetics dependent upon the drug and dosage formulation (1). This therefore allows one to extrapolate darkening data from accelerated studies back to room temperature long term studies.

Considerable research has also been devoted into the quantification of color fading by several investigators (2), (3), (4). Using reflectance color measurements, it has been shown to be possible to project the extent of color fading over time. One difficulty in electronic monitoring of color changes has been that apparent color changes can be greatly effected by factors such as the gloss of the surface or the darkening of the tablet substrate. This has resulted in a rather slow acceptance of electronic measurement techniques and continued reliance on visual monitoring of gross appearance changes.

Similarly, other organoleptic properties such as odor and taste can be best evaluated through the senses of smell and taste by the investigator for large changes. For the detection of small changes, evaluation panels are often the only viable measurement technique.

3. Hardness

Most commercially available hardness testers commonly measure the crushing strength of a tablet. This becomes quite valuable as a stability monitoring tool because a change in crushing strength may be an indication that the tablet matrix has changed structure. This can often signal changes in disintegration and dissolution rates. The popularity of obtaining hardness values also stems from the ease and speed in which it can be measured.

One example of how a decrease in hardness can be used to detect potential problems occurred during the formulation of a tablet which contained polyethylene glycol 8000 and sodium lauryl sulfate. The manufacturing process called for dispersal of the drug in molten polyethylene glycol 8000 at a temperature of about 80 °C to 90 °C. As was discovered later when the sodium lauryl sulfate was incorporated in the molten polyethylene glycol-drug mixture, sufficient sulfuric acid was formed to slowly attack the polyethylene glycol which formed water. A decrease in tablet hardness was the first clue that something unusual was occurring.

Numerous literature references to various means of measuring hardness are available (5), (6), (7), (8), (9), (10). Perhaps the method which has gained the greatest popularity and acceptance has been the Heberlein or Schleuniger type of hardness tester. One of the limitations of this type of hardness tester has been that for extremely hard tablets, the 20 Kg. force scale is often not sufficient. Recently, electronic hardness testers have become available with scales up to 50 Kg. This factor in combination with the improved mobility and lower maintenance of the electronic testers may eventually result in a transition away from the traditional Heberlein testers.

Hardness determinations can sometimes provide clues to potential problems of lamination or capping in tablets. The way in which a tablet fractures during hardness testing can aid a researcher in determining the weak points of a compressed tablet. The bonding and compressional forces within a tablet are often quite different dependent upon tablet shape and applied pressure. Weak points within a tablet can be exaggerated by accelerated stability conditions. For these reasons a researcher should look both at the actual hardness values but also the way in which a tablet breaks.

In order for hardness values to be of maximum use, a researcher must compare changes in hardness to disintegration and dissolution results. Hardness values by themselves are somewhat meaningless unless they can be used to guide additional testing.

4. Retained moisture

A physical test which I have found to be useful in evaluating new formulations and packaging materials has been retained moisture. For those drugs which are known to be moisture sensitive, this is particularly true.

As discussed previously, tablet hardness results can be evaluated only after one understands the meaning of the changes. It has been observed that hardness changes may be due to moisture loss or gain from the tablet especially when one is evaluating non-moisture barrier packaging such as PVC blisters. In instances where one observes a hardness increase in PVC blister packaged tablets stored at elevated temperatures but no change in tablets packaged in glass bottles, the usual cause is moisture loss form the tablets packaged in PVC blisters. This can be misleading as one may never see a loss of moisture and subsequent tablet hardening at normal room temperature and humidities. This can make extrapolations impossible and accelerated testing meaningless. A measurement of residual tablet moisture should aid in an investigator's interpretation of accelerated stability results.

Equilibrium moisture levels can also be used as a preformulation tool to avoid the creation of moisture sensitive products. In a test we commonly use in our laboratory, unpackaged tablets are stored in an open container at 25 °C and 50% R.H. After about one week of equilibration, the tablets are placed at 30 °C and 75% R.H. and the weight gain of the tablets is monitored for approximately ten days or until an equilibrium weight is reached. Most tablets reach equilibrium in about three days.

As a general rule, drugs which are known to be moisture sensitive should be formulated into a tablet which gains less than 1% moisture by weight. Depending upon the degree of sensitivity of the drug to moisture, a 2% weight gain may be acceptable. Only drugs which are known to be stable toward moisture should be formulated where greater than a 2% weight gain is obtained.

In those instances where one must formulate moisture sensitive drugs into a greater than 2% moisture weight gain base, protective packaging will most probably be necessary. While protective packaging can help, it merely retards the time of reaching equilibrium. One can expect that the stability of moisture sensitive products will become increasingly worse over time and the extrapolation of short term room temperature and accelerated data should be done with caution for setting expiration dates for humid climates.

Numerous techniques are available for the measurement of moisture in powders. Each of the various techniques has advantages and disadvantages over the other methods. Normally one must trade accuracy for speed. Based upon our experience we have found moisture loss upon heating values to be the most related to stability. This measurement of "free" or "non-bound" water in powders should be followed closely to help predict stability problems and to help interpret other data.

To help correlate data from one instrument to another we have used a common calibration test. An inert carrier such as dry sea sand is used. A quantitative amount of water is added using a syringe into the sea sand. The amount of water recovered compared to the amount added should be close to unity. While this simple test doesn't guarantee correlation of data obtained using different instruments, a lack of recovery of the added water should cause one to investigate further.

Another stability factor related to tablet moisture is pH. As moisture levels within a tablet increase, more drug can exist in a solubilized form and be subject to the internal pH environment of the tablet (11). Sometimes the moisture effect on a particular tablet can be minimized by optimizing the internal pH of the tablet, particularly for pH sensitive drugs. We commonly measure the pH of a 10% suspension or solution of ground tablets in distilled water over the time course of a stability study.

5. Disintegration

For the most part, disintegration tests are conducted because they have always been performed in the past. The importance of disintegration results has been eclipsed by dissolution testing. However, in those instances where disintegration has been shown to be the rate determining step in dissolution, disintegration can be a rapid and easily conducted meaningful test.

The equipment used for disintegration testing has become standardized over the years such that little difference exists worldwide. The possible exception to this are modifications made to the equipment to assist in end-point detection.

Perhaps the largest source of error in disintegration measurements is in the consistency of monitoring the end-point. Equipment has become commercially available within the past few years which provides for the disintegration end-points to be monitored electronically. While the electronic equipment does reduce the subjective evaluation of the disintegration end-point, the use of disks in the process becomes mandatory as the disks are part of the electronic detection system.

One area in which disintegration testing is still a procedure of choice would be in the evaluation of enteric films. Because the conditions in a disintegration process are normally more severe than in dissolution process, disintegration allows for a rapid evaluation of the integrity of an enteric coating. When placed in 0.1 N hydrochloric acid, a tablet with an imperfect enteric coating will be effected within a matter of minutes while intact enteric coated tablets should remain unchanged for one or two hours. For this type of evaluation, disks should not be used.

6. Dissolution

Dissolution testing has grown over the past decade to become one of the most widely accepted standards for the quality of a solid dosage form. In practice, dissolution testing measures the rate and extent of a drug dissolved in an *in vitro* system. The real strength of dissolution testing comes from a correlation of the *in vitro* results with *in vivo* data. The challenge that a pharmaceutical researcher must meet is that the dissolution procedure is designed to measure the release of drug from the dosage form without introducing an artificial hindrance or assistance.

The literature is filled with dissolution studies using various *in vitro* dissolution procedures and pieces of equipment. Over the years, two methods have more or less been adopted in the U.S. as the standard for dissolution procedures, the USP rotating basket and USP rotating paddle (12). While these two methods are certainly not the best procedures in every case, their use has been encouraged in the US in an attempt to standardize results and procedures between laboratories.

Of the two methods the USP rotating basket is probably the most prone to yield erroneous results due to artificial hindrances. One of the largest sources of error in the rotating basket method can come from poor uniformity of the media due to poor mixing of the solution. This can make results very dependent upon the place of sampling.

Another relatively common source of error can come from partial blockage of the openings in the basket mesh. Film coatings can sometimes cause this blockage particularly after they have become hydrated by storage under humid conditions. Gelatin from capsule dosage forms or from some sustained release formulations can also result in partial blockages.

An additional potential source of error for the USP rotating basket can come when a rapidly disintegrating tablet is evaluated. In those cases where the drug is poorly soluble, rapidly disintegrating tablets can release the particles of drug sufficiently fast that the drug particles can fall through the rotating basket screen and settle unmixed to the bottom of the dissolution vessel.

The USP rotating paddle method can also yield erroneous results due to procedural hindrances. However, for the most part, the rotating paddle method is superior to the USP rotating basket. In one particular instance in the evaluation of a buffered aspirin tablet, the buffering layer of the tablet disintegrated very quickly and covered the dissolving aspirin. Greatly different results could be obtained dependent upon whether the tablet was placed with the buffer layer facing up or down. This physical hindrance was resolved by increasing the rotational speed of the paddle sufficiently to eliminate the hydrophobic layer of buffering agents over the aspirin layer.

Modified release or controlled release dosage forms can pose very unusual problems for obtaining accurate dissolution results. Because most of these forms use hydrophobic materials to alter the dissolution of the drug substances, results can be greatly influenced by these materials. For example, many matrix release tablets will float after a portion of drug has been released. This requires that the tablet be held in place with a loose coil or wire.

Certain types of polymer coating materials can become sticky under heat or humidity stress. Particularly in coated bead or pellet forms, the pellets can fuse together to form a mass. This mass of pellets can result in a slower rate of dissolution if the mass stays intact. If the mass is artificially broken apart, a faster than anticipated dissolution rate can result if the integrity of the retardant coating is disrupted.

Enteric polymers pose a special challenge for dissolution testing because the pH of the media must be altered during the dissolution procedure. With the USP rotating basket and rotating paddle procedures a gradual pH transition is difficult. A procedure with which we have some success has been a flow cell technique in which the tablet or capsule is suspended in a bed of glass beads and the dissolution media is pumped across the dosage form. Unfortunately, the flow cell technique has not gained wide spread acceptance in the U.S. as have the two USP procedures.

In the final analysis one must rely on scientific observations while performing dissolution testing to try to identify potential sources of bias. Perhaps the best measure of a successful *in vitro* dissolution procedure is an *in vivo-in vitro* correlation. This not only can validate the method which was chosen, but also provide some idea of the significance of the *in vitro* data for establishing ranges of acceptability.

7. Conclusions

In summary, accelerated stability trials for evaluating the physico-chemical properties of solid dosage forms can provide very valuable information. However, a researcher must understand the drug with which he is working. He must realize that no single test or piece of information by itself is sufficient to base conclusions of the stability of a dosage form.

References

(1) Carstensen, J. T., Johnson, J. B., Valentine, W., and Vance, J. J., *J. Pharm. Sci, 53*, 1050 (1964).
(2) Hunter, R. S., "The Measurement of Appearance", John Wiley & Sons, Inc., New York, New York (1975).
(3) Everhard, M. E. and Goodhart, F. W., *J. Pharm. Sci, 52*, 281 (1963).
(4) Kubelka, P., *J. Optical Society America, 38*, 448 (1948).
(5) J. A. Hersey, *Manuf. Chem., 32*, Feb. (1969).
(6) J. Hasegawa, *J. Pharm. Soc. Japan, 75*, 480 (1955).
(7) D. B. Bock and K. Marshall, *J. Pharm. Sci., 57*, 481 (1968).
(8) H. J. Fairchild and F. Michel, *J. Pharm. Sic., 50*, 966 (1961).
(9) A. McCallum, J. Buchter and R. Albrecit, *J. Am. Pharm. Ass. Sci. Ed., 44*, 83 (1955).
(10) E. G. E. Shaper, E. G. Wolish and C. E. Engel, *J. Am. Pharm. Ass. Sci. Ed., 45*, 114 (1958).
(11) Carstensen, J. T., "Pharmaceutics of Solids and Solid Dosage Forms", John Wiley & Sons, Inc., New York, New York (1977).
(12) "The United States Pharmacopeia" 21st revision, Rockville, MD, United States Pharmacopeial Convention (1985), pp. 1243–1244.

IV. Changes in medicinal products and the consequences for their therapeutic application

A. Verain, D. Chulia, Faculté de Pharmacie, Université de Grenoble, F-Meylan Grenoble

1. Introduction

The topic seems a wager because it deals with stability.

In our universe, no example of stability can be found: everything changes, everything is transformed, everything evolves. We are thus living in a permanent state of instability, one in which the time factor is essential because these changes can be ultra slow, such as in rocks for instance; they can be slow, such as the ageing of our skin, or again they can be fast such as the volatilization of ether.

Therefore, what we must keep in mind is the concept of rate of transformation.

In the same way, when we deal with drugs and their stability, we must investigate the origin of their instability and its effects on their toxicologic and therapeutic activity. Kinetics of transformations of the various molecules present will be exhibited, whether it be physical, chemical or even technological transformations.

Therefore, the notion of drug stability covers a complex system which may be in equilibrium or not with its environment.

But, at the start of this paper, two points must be taken into account:

– Analysis, which makes it possible to detect transformations. Indeed some products, which seem stable when simple techniques are used, have been found to undergo transformations when current high technology is used. We are thus in a complexe domain where results can be affected by technology.
– Can pharmacological vigilance, which aims at following the changes occurring in the life of drugs, give use dangerous examples of instability? The answer is NO, despite the great instability of our therapeutically active molecules, despite incompatibilities likely to appear as time goes by. One of the aims of this paper will be to answer this question.

2. Notion of Stability

A drug is an association of one or more active principles and one or more excipients intended to produce the final and permanent dosage form adapted to the end-use of this drug.

When this drug is being manufactured, the various components have a certain internal energy and a certain reactivity. It is thus possible to define an entropy for each component, this entropy being known only to within a constant factor.

This system is not isolated; it is subjected to various possible actions from the outside environment:

Physical: – temperature
                 – pressure
                 – humidity
                 – radiation
Chemical: – action of oxygen
                 – action of water, acids, bases

Under these various energy-carrying influences, drugs will alter more or less rapidly, which may entail a modification in their toxicology-pharmacological activity.

This alteration can affect active principles through a split in molecules which will cause the appearance of new molecules that may be more or less active than the original substance. In this case, we are dealing with a degradation. This change can only occur with a reduction in free energy and, therefore, an increase in entropy.

Excipients, which are chemical bodies, are apt to react and are not neutral as has so often been thought. So, the modification of active molecules can also be caused by a reaction with an excipient. A new substance is thus created with properties likely to be different from those of the original molecule.

Also, there is a substantial quantity of excipients in drugs and, therefore, they may also react against the physical and chemical aggressions of the environment and may alter either by decaying, converting or reacting.

It is virtually certain that these transformations take place spontaneously, but the rate at which new molecules are formed must be very low; indeed the ageing of a drug is linked to this rate.

A drug will be regarded as aged and therefore unfit for consumption, when a given fraction of the initial molecules has disappeared.

In order to see what is tolerable and try to know the newly-formed bodies, accelerated ageing methods are used, mainly by increasing the action of physical agents that is temperature, radiation, humidity.

In drugs, transformations due to ageing are irreversible, but since they consist of a succession of states of near-equilibrium (that is, very slow transformation), it should be possible to define the entropy of the system by measuring the quantity of heat exchanged and the temperature.

It would thus be possible to note that the entropy of drugs (that is the sum of the entropies of active principles and excipients), increases as time goes by, thereby showing a loss of free energy. Indeed, the useful of free energy is equal to the difference between the internal energy U (fixed from the outset) and the product of the entropy S by the thermodynamic temperature.

$$\Psi = U - TS$$

Since S increases spontaneously and T is constant, the value of Ψ decreases with time. Nevertheless, for the reaction (that is to say the alteration) to take place, and thus for S to increase, the quantity of emitted heat during the transformation must be positive, that is, the reaction must be exothermic according to Berthelot's equation. If it is endothermic, the reaction is impossible, or, at least, very unlikely to take place.

Research should be carried out in this field in order to block reactions between active principles and excipients.

This leads us to look into the subject of reactivity, whether it be between constituents or even of each element affected by external factors.

This reactivity will determine the stability of the product which can be regarded as an artificial system with a thermodynamic equilibrium and a potential of interactions between ions present.

This is an extremely complex problem because:

– active principles may decay and convert to substances apt to react with each other,
– excipients are apt to exhibit the same drawbacks,
– these two categories of substances may react with each other,
– measuring and identifying the quantity of substances produced after a relatively short period of time is not always possible.

For the evaluation the Arrhenius equation is applied which relates the reaction rate k to the activation energy E. Furthermore the variation in temperature ΔT is linearly dependent upon the number of molecules formed and upon the variation in the enthalpy of the system.

Whereas variations in temperature can be easily measured, such is not the case for the variation rate and above all for the enthalpy variation. At the very most, only an order of magnitude can be arrived at.

These general considerations show that empirical methods to assess ageing processes (whether it be normal or accelerated) are still the only ones giving some information, especially if the rules to use them are well-defined.

3. Stability and Production

In this discussion products of biological origin (vegetal, animal, bacterial) which constitute complex systems where many physical, chemical and, especially, biological transformations take place (well known activity losses) will be left aside. The example of vaccines has often been mentioned.

Therefore the discussion will be focused on chemical molecules, therapeutically active, which means that they are reactive and decay rapidly when isolated, hence problems of preserving and storing raw materials.

This is where industrial pharmacy comes in. Its aim is to devise and manufacture medicines, that means, to place a degradable molecule in a medium that will stabilise it for three to five years, for the medicines shelf life.

To find the means to stabilise the molecule, its properties and degradation products must be perfectly known. This is the information required in the dossier of application of Marketing Permission in France, especially in the Scientific Report.

It is therefore with full knowledge of the requirements that the pharmaceutical manufacturer will develop his formulation and stabilise the molecules already known to be rather unstable.

In this context Professor Dufraisse should be quoted about this subject:

"Do not be afraid of learning too much about the material you are dealing with, do not have any scruples, you may resort to any method to question it. Not a single one is illicit, perfidious or even simply indiscreet."

The first step will be to see how to create such a favourable medium, this is the object of formulation.

Then the variations will be studied this system may undergo during the manufacturing process.

3.1 The Formulation Process

The formulator will try and find a form which enables the active principle to have the greatest possible effect at the right place and time.

When tablet formulas are developed in which 10% of the active principle are bioavailable, there are reasons to be flabbergasted!

Moreover, the selected dosage form will stabilise the active principle by protecting it, depending on circumstances, from air, light, heat and humidity, but also by avoiding incompatibilities occurring either with other active principles or with excipients. Without such precautions, the formulation would be a regression, not an improvement.

In order to obtain a good formulation, it is essential that the raw material should be well-known, and more expecially the active molecule. That is all its structural changes (such as polymorphism, isomerisation, inversion), its reactivity and its sensibility to humidity should be well-known.

3.1.1 Structural Changes

3.1.1.1 Polymorphism

Today, the formulator cannot ignore the polymorphic nature of the molecule he is handling, whether it be an active principle or an excipient. Each crystalline form of a molecule has its own thermodynamic and stability characteristics which may influence the biological activity of the molecule. As a rule, the most thermodynamically unstable form is the most active because it is the most soluble one.

Therefore, the formulator must carefully choose the right polymorph and see to it that it will not alter during the whole preservation period.

Examples:

- Novobiocin is marketed as a suspension in its therapeutically active amorphous acidic form. But in less than six months, at room temperature, it converts to a much less soluble crystalline form.
- Choramphenicol exists as a stearate and as a palmitate both present three forms:
  - a non-active crystalline form A
  - an active crystalline form B
  - an active amorphe form C

These three forms differ from one another by their X-ray and infra-red diffraction spectra. Forms B and C are obviously the only ones that are to be used. Indeed the American FDA stipulates that the stearate chloramphènicol syrup should not contain more than 10% of polymorph A. Besides, the formulator knows that in order to stabilise chloramphenicol palmitate, he needs only to add to the preparation some stearate which will convert, leaving the palmitate intact.

- In the same way sodium cholate is used to stabilise cholesterol
- hydrocortisone is used to stabilise cortisone acetate.

- Sulfathiazole converts under the effect of a rise in temperature.
  Wurster and Hankell observed changes in crystalline forms during the compressions, a conversion probably due to freed adiabatic heat.
- Sulfametoxydiazine passes from polymorph 1 to polymorph 2 as temperature increases. This reaction is even faster in the presence of water vapour since the compound is recrystallised on the surface.

But the formulator knows that some polymorphic changes can be considerably retarded simply by dehydrating the molecule environment (the excipient for instance), or again by using some macromolecules that will be adsorbed on the surface of the crystal in transformation and block the latter. Thus sodium carboxymethyl cellulose, pectin, gum arabic and gelatin inhibit the conversion of the beta form of chlortetracycline hydrochloride. PVP inhibits the crystallisation of amorphous nabilone. In the latter case the hypothesis put forward is that hydrogen bonds established between nabilone and the polymer block intermolecular hydrogen reactions which are necessary to crystallisation.

3.1.1.2 Isomerisation

Many conversion of product A into B are catalysed by heat or light. Wellknown examples are mannitol, vitamin D_2 and Hyosciamine L. The epimerisation of lactam antibiotics leads to various compounds and, therefore, different activities. Prostaglandins are more stable in a liquid system than in a solid one, because the tendency to isomerisation is stronger in the solid state.

3.1.1.3 Inversion

As regards optical inversions, biochemists have established earlier that the natural active forms of amino-acids were the levorotatory ones. The same was true for compounds, such as adrenaline, whose racemic form was 20 times less active than the levorotatory form. Thanks to PASTEUR, it was possible to separate and utilise the active compound via adrenaline tartrate.

As for Ethambutol, scientific literature shows that the levorotatory form of ethambutol is 14 times as active as the the the racemic one.

Formerly, such preparations would exhibit unexplained losses of activity. Today, the formulator must know right from the start the structural changes that can take place within a molecule. As a result, he must chose the most active form and follow up its evolution thanks to a simple method such as dissolution kinetics which will evince any change in the solubility of the product.

3.1.2 Reactivity

Knowing the reaction mechanism of the product present, the formulator has several means of controlling highly reactive molecules.

Technological aids:

– coating of oxidisable molecules such as vitamin C or hydrolysable ones such as aspirin
– nebulizing emulsions in order to reestablish a balance between the components
– adding stabilising agents, for instance sodium metabisulfite to block the conversion of adrenaline into adrenochrome; sodium bisulfite is used to block the conversion of morphine into pseudomorphine.

3.1.3 Sensibility to Humidity

The hygroscopy of a molecule must be established from the start of a study in order to take all required protective measures such as the use of air-tight packaging or controlled atmosphere rooms. To do so, the sorption and desorption curves in a humidity-controlled atmosphere must be known.

A good example of this is the hydrolysis of vitamin A contained in a multivitamin preparation.

Small quantities of water may sometimes have a negative effect.

If in a 300 mg tablet there are 5.6 mg of an active product whose molecular weight is 140 and 0.18% humidity, the latter seems unimportant. However, calculations show that the tablet contains:

$$\frac{516}{140} = 0.04 \text{ milliequivalents of active product}$$

and

$$\frac{0.18 \times 300}{100 \times 18} = 0.03 \text{ milliequivalents of water}$$

Therefore hydrolysis of the active product may well take place if it exhibits ester or amide bonds. Now, it must kept in mind that the starch introduced into the formula contains from 10% to 20% of water.

Likewise, in thiamine hydrochlorate and microcrystalline cellulose tablets the reaction is much greater in the presence of water.

Therefore, starting from an unstable molecule, the formulator will create a stable drug, but it should be added: "stable under perfect-well stipulated conditions".

Hence the important role of packaging which, thanks to a perfectly adapted material, allows the drug to be protected and stored in a suitable environment of temperature, humidity and air (oxygen). Thus insulin is tube stored at $+4°C$.

It is worth mentioning that new molecules are more and more fragile and more and more sensitive, so that refrigerators and even deep-freezers are now necessary in chemists' shops. This is the reason why in the pharmaceutical dossier stability tests are required. Their positive results show that the formulator has chosen the right excipients and/or the right sort of packaging.

3.2 Production

If a formulation is not perfectly observed during production, there will be no conformity, hence incidents and lower therapeutic potency. This is the clue to therapeutic troubles.

3.2.1 Polymorphism

Indeed, during a given operation, or faulty storage, the active product may have re-crystallised into another form. One example is the use of a new type of crusher to manufacture digoxin which turned the crystallised form into the more soluble amorphous form, hence greater plasmatic concentrations and the occurrence of therapeutic. incidents.

During a granulation process the active product may recrystallise.

Finally, during mixing or crushing operations, crystals may be altered and faulty crystals may be generated.

In the dry state, under the effect of other constituents of the dosage form, or the action of traces of remaining solvent or some impurities, the selected crystalline form may change slowly during storage. Thus corticoïds exhibit 5 or 6 different crystalline forms and some cortisone acetate preparations have undergone substantial decreases in activity.

In like manner, a lyophilisation operation can insidiously generate crystalline changes or different ratios between crystalline products and amorphous products.

Bogardus reports that after the heating stage of lyophilisation he found 4 different polymorphs of sodium nafcillin. Likewise, sodium cephalothin exhibited various percentages of crystalline forms depending on the humidity content (0 to 31%).

3.2.2 Reactivity

For instance, steroid preparations were oxidised by air, the phenolic function of a steroid having converted to a ketonic function, hence a difference in activity.

Unforeseen temperature rises or due to the higher speed of some machine may induce faster kinetics, hence degradations or reactions. Thus addition reaction may occur: for instance, benzocaïne is deactivated by the glucose used as a granulating agent because a Benzocaïne N glucoside is formed.

In the same way, a Maillard reaction between oses and amines may be triggered; once started a self-catalysing process leads to the formation of an inactive complex.

Another mishap is the reaction between lactose and a amine chloride in the presence of a basic lubricant.

To give a further example, it can be said that isoniazid and lactose also react to produce a browning isonicotinoyl hydrazone of lactose hydroxymethylfurfural. Dextroamphetamine sulfate also reacts with lactose. In the presence of hydroxy-methylfurfural, a browning reaction makes haloperidol inactive. Yet lactose is one of our major excipients and performs well if manufacturing processes are well-controlled.

The same kind of reactions are to be found when amines react with β-cyclodextrin or desoxycholic acid and fatty acid derivatives with cyclodextrins. In all these cases, inactive products are obtained.

Exchange reactions may also take place:

for instance A + BC yielding AB + C
                    or
              AB + CD yielding AD + BC

for instance, the exchange reaction of aspirin with phenylephrine resulting in the loss of activity of the latter product.

A transacetylation is reported to explain the degradatation of codeineaspirin tablets; whereas there is no exchange if aspirin and acetaminophen are mixed.

Still talking about aspirin, in the presence of calcium stearate this molecule yields calcium acetylsalicynate which is destabilised and the molecule is broken down.

3.2.3 Humidity

One important factor, not depending on formulation, is the humidity contained in manufacturing laboratories.

Any variation in the relative humidity is conducive to the hydrolysis of active principles. This takes place with penicillin, aspirin, atropine and multivitamin tablets for which slight variations in the water content have resulted in a degradation of vitamins A and D. The same phenomenon has been reported for cellulose-based thiamine hydrochloride tablets.

This humidity, even at a normal percentage, can be adsorbed whenever new surfaces are bound either by heating, compression or grinding. For instance, some accidents have been caused by lactose monohydrate freeing one water molecule at the time of grinding.

3.2.4 Mechanical Manipulation

Any slight and involuntary variation during a fabrication operation may cause problems.

For instance, depending on the lyophilisation process, diverse behaviours of the product may be induced. The stability of prasterone sulfate (a steroid used in obstetrics) is increased if polyvinylpyrrolidone (PVP) or glycine have been used as additives to the lyophilising medium, if not, an inactive product is reconstituted. Another such example is the stabilisation of piperazylphenylbenzofuran (an antiviral substance) by the addition of isopropanol in the buffered drug solution.

4. Medicinal accidents due to faulty fabrication techniques or instabilities

In this part examples are given of medicinal accidents caused by faulty fabrication techniques and/or changes occurring in the final dosage form and which affected patients.

Accidents noted above resulting from research in the development laboratories have led to drastic laws that have prevented in the past few years (and should prevent in the future) the occurrence of incidents.

Unfortunately, errare humanum est!

It should be added that if changes in therapeutic activity and the emergence of toxicity are rare, the breakdown of therapeutic potency may be extremely serious as a patient suffering from a serious disease may not be treated and thus suffer from the consequences.

4.1 Incidents independent of the chemical structure of the active molecule

– At the final dosage form stage, oesophagites have been reported to be due to an increase in the "hardening" of tablets with time. The same phenomenon occurs with tablets that are too large and capsules that stick to the oesophageal wall in 8 to 20% of the cases.

In case of prolonged stagnation, these forms will release their active principle and, if the latter causes irritation, serious incidents will arise, in particular ulcerations and perforations whose prognosis may be gloomy.

– Tablets that had hardened during storage have been found in faeces. Such was the case with the mixture aspirin-tricalcium phosphate.

The damage, however, can be even more serious: a number of patients have had painful spasms or intestinal obstruction.

– Granulometry may also evolve, in spite of it being determined at the time of formulation.

– Particles of griseofulvin, whose powder had been micronized in order to improve bioavailability, clustered again in the suspension so that bioavailability was substantially diminished.

– Numerous incidents due to packaging have also been reported. When they can be spotted early, this is not very serious because the manufacturing of the pharmaceutical can be stopped.

The migration of the active principle into the plastic structure of pharmaceutical packaging may be observed:

● a polyethylene tube containing a salicylic acid ointment had its outer surface covered with salicyclic acid crystals.

● the same thing happened with a polyethylene film that contained aspirin.

● a mixture of vitamin B migrated into the wall of a polyethylene vial.

● a hexachlorophene-based eye-lotion became too concentrated after the water had evaporated through the wall of a plastic vial: the patient's eye was burnt.

● human blood that had been preserved at $+4\,°C$ in a plastic vial containing 10 milligrams of plasticizer. Twenty-one days later, the 10 mg of plasticizer were found in the lipoproteinic part of the plasma.

● a PVC vial incorporating -2-ethyl-hexylphtalate used as a plasticizer, was filled with bovine albumin; the latter extracted most of the plasticizer, that was found in the abdominal fat of two patients that had be given the product.

Since two-way migrations in a plastic container were evidenced, container-contents reactions have been required in the application dossier for Marketing Permission in France. Professor PELLERIN has become one of the specialists in this area, which is extremely important, given the vast number of plastic materials used nowadays.

– Another example is the known adsorbent power of bentonite, plastics, rubber, which, in multidose vials, caused the antiseptics present to disappear, which brought about an increase in bacteria in the preparations.

This is the reason why, the potency of the preparation of the end of the shelf life is now required information.

– Manufacturers have had trouble with prednisolone, phenylbutazone, and chloramphenicol tablets because the excipients chosen were not sufficiently porous, hence an excessive increase in the dissolution rate, so that, once more there was no bioavailability.

– During sterilization of buffered chloramphenicol the concentration in OH ions being 110 times higher at $120\,°C$ than at $20\,°C$, the active principle was inhibited. The same thing occurred for streptomycine in a Sorensen solution.

4.2 Incidents related to the active molecule

Scientific literature mentions few cases, and the recently introduced pharmacovigilance service has not yet reported a single accident resulting from a change in the active molecule in a preparation. This is due to the precautions taken but also to a well-known chemical fact: degradation compounds of a molecule are, in most cases, less reactive, therefore less toxic. This is essential.

Generally speaking we may be confronted:

- either with an increase in toxicity,
- or with an exacerbation of the therapeutic potency, a decrease, or even its disappearance.

Two well known examples should be given due to increased toxicity:

- Di-iodo-diethylethane or Stalinon introduced into France in 1953 brought about a real disaster due to the formation of tri-iodo-ethylethane and above all of mono-iodo-diethylethane. Indeed, 270 people suffering from furunculosis or acne and treated with the product were proved to have been poisoned. 101 of them died. This intoxication went through several phases:
  - a phase of latency lasting several days,
  - strong and lasting headaches,
  - a phase of functional disorders such as vomitting, photophobia, dizziness,
  - general signs: hypothermia, bradycardia, rapid loss of weight, alterations in psyche,
  - and neurological disorders: convulsions, meningitis.

The disease evolves to death which occurs after a coma or again after a heart or respiratory failure. The clinical symptoms are similar to those of a meningeal cerebro-medullar oedema.

- Elixir Masengil containing a sulfamide base in a solution of di-ethylene glycol, the toxicity of glycol certainly played its part, but so did that of the product generated by the sulfamide-glycol interaction. All the patients that drank that elixir died, and the manufacturer committed suicide.

  It was after those incidents that the Ministry of Health required toxicological test records and more advanced testing of the dosage form.
- Nephrotoxicity accidents caused by tetracycline are in fact due to di-hydro-tetracycline that developed with time.
- PAS used to be toxic because it produced metaaminophenol in the human body.
- Allergic accidents due to the parent molecule: penicillin or its degradation products.

  Harmful reactions due to intravenous injections of Penicillin G have been reported. These reactions are not attributable to the product itself because newly-manufactured preparations do not cause them, but probably to degradation products that have not yet been identified.

In the first case, accidents consisted in haemolytic anaemia and neutropenia, whereas none of these harmful effects are produced in the second group.

- Ioniazid is hepato-toxic. About 10% of patients who are given Rimifon show an increase in the quality of transaminases due to an isoniazid metabolite. Isoniazid inductors increase the concentration in metabolites, hence the cases of acute hepatitis reported. One of the inductors not to be associated with isoniazid in the same preparation is rifampicin neither are anaesthetics, or, perhaps, inductor excipients.
- Preparations containing hydrochlorothiazide and potassium chloride produced ulcers resulting in the patients's death. The ulcers were formulation-dependent and lipophilic matrices which do not adhere to the mucin wall solved the problem. The same accidents happened with the new "Oros" dosage form.
- Stored chlorhexidine-based preparations may evolve to the formation of para-chloraniline (PCA). The maximum allowed content of PCA is 500 ppm in view of its toxicity. But in ill-preserved preparations concentration can reach 2000 ppm, which has been the cause of accidents.
- Halothane or 2-bromo-2 chloro-1-1-1 trifluorethane ($C_2HBrClF_3$) is an anaesthetic, that caused hepatic lesions in Europe as well as in the USA when it contained 0.02% dichlorohexafluorobutene.

Conversely, there can be a loss in toxicity: such is the case for phenacetin whose therapeutic potency is chiefly due to its metabolite, paracetamol. The latter is less toxic, hence its use nowadays.

The therapeutic potency of a drug product may disappear when the active product is broken down by degradation reactions (hydrolysis, oxidation). Many examples have been observed in medical centres: penicillin, adrenaline, atropine. Rifampicin also generates many metabolites, but all are non-toxic and are as potent as rifampicin itself. On the other hand, when the derivative (which is also non-toxic) is formed, there is a general decrease in the potency of the preparation.

Among cases where a change in therapeutic activity occurs, aspirin, is also an example that can be analysed:

acetylsalicylic acid → salicylic acid

Both compounds produce ulcers, aspirin because it is anti-prostaglandin, salicylic acid because of its acidity, but aspirin is analgetic and antipyretic whereas salicyclic acid is anti-inflammatory and keratolytic.

Certainly, there are other instances and it should be continued to review them for a future conference.

5. Conclusions

At the end of this paper, where only few actual examples have been given, it appears that the active molecule, which is a source of changes and metabolisation, is very different from the drug developed by the formulator. Such development is difficult and complex, and requires making many choices that will prevent, as often as possible, harmful effects of the molecule. Formulation has a considerable biological influence on the molecule. So we must be careful in the development of medicines which are a source of health necessary to all of us. The future will belong to the new pharmaceutical forms such as nano-capsules and liposomes which will carry drugs at the desired moment to the places where they are needed; it must also be added the DNA carrying agent, grooved and filled red blood corpuscules and magnetic macromolecules which will all ensure low toxicity in view of the small amount of molecules introduced into the body.

V. Japanese Guideline for Stability Testing

T. Nagai, Department of Pharmaceutics, Hoshi University, Tokyo/Japan

1. Introduction

General view regarding the approval of applications of new drugs in Japan.

The regulations regarding the approval of applications of new drugs often cause distressing problems not only for manufacturers or importers in Japan but also for foreign pharmaceutical companies who wish to export their products to Japan. It was often mentioned that troubles arise between the staff of non-Japanese parent companies headquartered overseas and their branch offices in Japan, in understanding the Japanese regulatory system of approval; these misunderstandings may have been due not only to linguistic difficulties hampering communication but also to an inability to understand the differences in the systems.

In the past, before the GLP and GMP were established, the regulating Japanese authorities did not accept data compiled in foreign countries. This may have been reasonable from both scientific and political viewpoints, and was not enforced to protect domestic Japanese pharmaceutical companies in competition with foreign ones. Considering the circumstances surrounding Japan, dual attitudes prevailed.

The idea that we should be fair in accepting foreign data even if it was compiled abroad was countered with the thought that we should be fair in not accepting it, too. This duality created dissatisfaction amongst the staff and management of foreign companies, especially from advanced nations.

However, the situation has greatly changed since the GLP and other relevant guidelines were established to assure first of all the safety of drugs, and in part to solve the present problem of trading-conflict between Japan and other nations. Now, almost all data (except for clinical trials) are said to be accepted, if they are compiled following the above-mentioned Japanese guidelines. These circumstances may expand to those of clinical trials, as the so-called GCP, (a guideline for practice in clinical trials), has recently been established.

The personal past experience of the author (serving the Ministry of Health and Welfare as a member of both the Subcommittee on New Drugs and the Subcommittee on Combination Drugs), prompts him to say that even data which has been compiled without following the Japanese guidelines exactly might be accepted, if there are no problems in the reasoning logic of it, indicating an equivalency to data which might be compiled following the above-mentioned guidelines. However, many companies have preferred recompiling data following the Japanese guidelines to reviewing inconsistencies in "reasoning" and "indicating," as difficulties might arise in the above-mentioned logic (reasoning).

A better understanding of the Japanese regulatory system for approval of pharmaceuticals might be helpful in solving potential problems businesses in Japan might face.

It will be attempted to show Japanese guidelines for stability testing as clearly as it can be from the authors experience. He would like to emphasize that he is not representing any Japanese regulatory authority but a participant from the academic side. Therefore, it would be appreciated if the Japanese authorities would be querried frankly concerning those matters which can not be explained here.

2. Cooperative investigation on the establishment of the method for stability test for pharmaceutical preparations

It may be difficult to find a completely general rule for stability test of drugs. However, we may find some general method for it. The request to establish it had arisen from both the regulatory and pharmaceutical industry sides in Japan. In 1977, Pharmaceutical Affairs Bureau of Ministry of Health and Welfare organized the Investigation Team on the Establishment of the Method for Stability Test for Pharmaceutical Preparations as the 3 years' project headed by Nagai myself. The investigation was carried out by 36 facilities (Hoshi University, National Institute of Hygienic Sciences and 34 pharmaceutical industries) using aspirin tablets and ascorbic acid powders as the test samples. The test was done at several temperatures and humidities, and for packed and non-packed samples. The amount of aspirin and the water content were determined for aspirin tablets and the change in color and the loss on drying for ascorbic acid powders.

Considering the result in a preliminary experiment, the experimental conditions were mainly set as follows:

- preservation conditions, temperature and humidity,
- items to measure (except for the drug content),
- packing materials and forms,
- determination of drug content (active ingredient only and no decomposed products),
- size of descicator,
- amount of sample and where to put it in a descicator,
- temperature deviation in thermostat,
- change in relative humidity due to sublimations (especially aspirin),
- frequency of measurements and control limit.

The results were published (1). Analyzing statistically, the expiration date till 90% drug content was estimated by Woolfe's (2) and Carstensen's equations (3). These results agreed well with the observed values at 25 °C. In the accelerated test, the estimated values obtained by the observation for 6 months was closer to the observed values than those done for 3 months. The results obtained at 40 °C, 75% R. H. for one month corresponded to those at 25 °C, 75% R. H. for about one year.

The above results were taken into consideration by the Ministry of Health and Welfare in the establishment of "Standards for stability testing of new drugs," which will be described later.

3. General matters concerning the data of stability testing to be submitted when applying for approval to manufacture (or import) new drugs

With regard to the handling of data on stability to be submitted in applying for manufacturing (or importing) approval of drugs in Japan, there have been issued a series of notifications from Pharmaceutical Affairs Bureau (or Evaluation and Registration Division of the Bureau) of the Ministry of Health and Welfare. Among them, the basic policy concerning the current guideline for stability testing is described in the notification issued on March 31, 1980 as "Standards for stability testing of new drugs." Additionally, it is reminded (June 8, 1984) that if there are proper reasons, some (or all) of the items in the standards mentioned above do not have to be always observed.

The following general matters are described in the notification concerning the data of stability testing to be submitted when applying for approval to manufacture (or import) new drugs, which was issued on March 31, 1980.

3.1. The stability test concerned shall be carried out at adequately equipped facilities by experienced researchers, in conformity with the "Standards for stability testing of new drugs", which will be described later in detail. The following shall be supplied when submitting test data:

3.1.1 Information about the facilities where the tests took place, i.e.,

● the name and address of the facilities
● the date of establishment
● the parent body
● the organization
● an outline of the equipments
  (such as their type and other relevant details)
● any other relevant informations.

3.1.2 Information about the researchers who are described in the research reports as having carried out the test concerned, i.e.,

- their personal histories
- background details of research work done in the past
- any other relevant informations.

3.2. All data shall be written in Japanese. If the materials is translated from a foreign language, a total translation shall be submitted as well as the original; in addition the names, titles and qualifications of both the translators involved and the technical personnel who finally examined the content shall be mentioned.

3.3 In the case of any materials being submitted which is based on tests carried out overseas, the contents of such foreign test shall meet Japanese standards. New drugs which are submitted for import approval accompanied by data from tests carried out overseas shall have already been given approval or permission over seas. All data on stability tests made available to the foreign authorities concerned at the time of approval of the drug shall be submitted, accompanied by a certificate from the relevant foreign government or organization that such data was taken into consideration at the time of granting approval.

3.4 Test records shall be preserved for a period of at least five years after the date of approval for manufacture (or import) of the drug concerned.

4. Standards for stability testing of new drugs (March 31, 1980)

The effect on stability of bulk powders and finished products shall be studied in all the possible conditions of handling. For example, for a drug to be stored in tight containers, change in stability with time under the effect of light, heat and temperature on exposure to air shall be studied. The same study is required in the test under severe conditions (severe test). At the same time, decomposition products shall be identified as precisely as possible and, if necessary, their toxicity and general pharmacology shall be investigated. In consideration of the results of the stability test in many directions, the best conditions of storage and reasonable expiration date shall be determined.

"Standards for stability testing of new drugs" (March 31, 1980) is described in detail as follows:

4.1 Stability tests of new drugs shall be carried out in conformity with the following.

4.1.1 The stability of a new drugs shall be investigated in both the long-term preservation test as defined under 4.2 below and the severe test as defined under 4.3 below.

4.1.2 The long-term preservation test shall be carried out by Method A (4.2.2.1 below) or Method B (4.2.2.2 below):

4.1.2.1 In case the Method A is employed, preservations such as temperature, humidity etc. must be recorded and described in the test results. If the preservation conditions are considered to differ extremely from the standard meteorological conditions in Japan, such test result shall not be accepted.

4.1.2.2 If the Method A is employed and if particular conditions are set concerning preservation conditions, or if a period for expiration is set, the ground for setting so shall be stated without fail.

4.1.2.3 If the approval for manufacture (or import) has been granted based on the results of the test performed by the Method B, the test for confirmation of stability as one of the measures for quality control shall be performed by the Method A after the start of manufacture (or import).

4.2 Long-term preservation test.

4.2.1 Purpose: This test is performed to ascertain whether the quality of the new drug is maintained during certain periods of distribution.

4.2.2 Methods etc.:

4.2.2.1 Method A.:

- Sample: the finished product (including bulk product in case the new drug contains a novel active ingredients
- Number of lots: 3 lots
- Preservation conditions: room temperature (or under the conditions specified as such, if particular conditions are set as a storage method in the application sheet for approval)
- Period: 3 years ore more (or the period specified as such or more, if the period for expiration is set in the application sheet for approval)
- Time of measurement: at the start of the test and regularly thereafter at the intervals not exceeding six months
- Contents of measurement: the items deemed necessary for quality control.
- Frequency of measurement: 3 times (however, the frequency may be reduced for some measurement items, depending on measurement variation, precision of the measurement method, etc.).

4.2.2.2 Method B.:

- Sample: the same as that under Method A
- Number of lots: the same as that under Method A

- Preservation conditions: 25 °C ($\pm$ 1 °C), 75% R.H. ($\pm$ 5%).
- Period: 2 years
- Measurement dates: at the start of the test and 3, 4, 9, 12, 18 and 24 months thereafter
- Contents of measurement: the same as those under Method A
- Frequency of measurement: the same as that under Method A.

4.3 Severe test.

4.3.1 Purpose: This test is performed to estimate the stability at room temperature and to investigate decomposed products.

4.3.2 Test conditions etc.:

4.3.2.1 The three conditions – light, temperature and humidity – shall be considered in setting the test conditions. As for the bulk substance, the test in aqueous solution shall, in principle, be included.

4.3.2.2 Decomposition products shall be identified; major decomposition products shall be tested for toxicity and pharmacology.

4.3.2.3 The test for ascertaining the absence of decomposition product shall be performed by chromatography or other suitable methods under three or more different conditions (comment: three or more different conditions of chromatography or three or more different test methods).

5 Accelerated test standards

This test is performed to estimate, by a short-term test, the quality of a drug in a certain period of distribution.

However, if, according to the comparison of the result with that under the storage conditions in the above "Standards for stability testing of new drugs" (March 31, 1980), this test is found not to serve the purpose of the test, and if a change in the sample with time may occur, the test described in the above "Standards" shall be performed.

When a partial modification of a finished product is intended, the result of relative comparative test of the finished product before and after the modification may be accepted. This relative comparative test shall be performed for three months or more, in principle, under 40 °C ($\pm$ 1 °), R.H. 75% ($\pm$ 5%), though the regular accelerated test in performed as in the following.

The regular method of the accelerated test is as follows:

- Sample: the finished product (including bulk product in case the new drug contains a novel active ingredients.
- Number of lots: 3 lots.
- Preservation conditions:
  - in principle, under 40 °C (± 1°), R.H. 75% ($\pm 5\%$)
  - room temperature (or under the conditions specified as such, in case particular conditions are set as a storage method in the application sheet for approval).
- Period: 6 months or more.
- Time of measurement: 4 times including the measurement at the start of the test.
- Contents of measurement: in principle, all the items indicated in the columns or 'specifications" and "test method" in the application form.
- Frequency of measurement: 3 times (however, the frequency may be reduced for some measurement items, depending on measurement variation, precision of the measurement method, etc.).

6. Additional guideline concerning the standards for stability testing of new drugs (June 8, 1984)

Concerning "Standards for stability testing of new drugs" (March 31, 1980), the following additional guideline has been given.

6.1 If there are proper reasons, some (or all) of the items in the standard do not have to be always observed.

6.2 For "new drugs containing a new active ingredients", etc. (the data of long-term storage test and severe test being requested for their application for approval), the application was formerly stipulated so far to be file after completion of the stability test. Now, in principle, if the product can be estimated to have a long-term stability on the basis of the results of severe test and accelerated test and if at the time of the application the effective period (shelf-life) of the drug can be tentatively set at one year or more on the basis of the long-term storage test carried out by method A, the application for approval shall be acceptable to be filed even while the long-term storage test are still under way. However, the final results of the continued and completed long-term storage test must be submitted prior to the of approval.

6.3 In the case of drugs with new active ingredients, etc., which have been jointly developed by more than one party (i.e., drugs covered by contracts providing for joint-ownership of the development materials, including the raw data, and the accumulated technologies and knowledge), if one of the developing parties carries out the long-term storage test and severe test require for filing of the application of approval, then, in principle, it shall be permissible for the other developing parties to substitute the performance of the accelerated test for the long-term storage test and the severe test in the Standards.

6.4 In the case of drug products which are provided as bulk products for use in the manufacture of other drugs, the following procedures shall be applied.

6.4.1 With regard to drug products containing a new active ingredient, if the manufacturing countries or manufacturing methods are more than one, it shall be permissible to carry out the long-term storage test and the severe test on any one of the drug products.

6.4.2 With regard to "the other drug products" (ethical and OTC me-too drugs), in principle, it shall not be necessary to submit the stability test data.

6.5 With regard to drug products other than the bulk drug products, the following procedures shall be applied.

6.5.1 If the manufacturing countries are more than one and if the packing materials and the packing forms are plural, each product shall be subjected to the tests in accordance with 6.5.1.1 and 6.5.1.2 below.

6.5.1.1 If the manufacturing countries are plural and if the drug product contains a new active ingredient, etc., the long-term storage test and the severe test shall be carried out on the product manufactured in any one of the manufacturing countries, and the products manufactured in the remaining countries shall, in principle, be subjected to the accelerated test. In the case of "the other drug products", each product shall be subjected to the accelerated test.

6.5.1.2 If the packing materials and the packing forms are plural for one finished and packed product (i.e., one packing material and one packing form) and if the drug product contains a new active ingredient, etc., the long term storage test and severe test shall be carried out, while "the other drug products" shall be subjected to the accelerated test. For the products with other packing materials and packing forms, in principle, the relative comparative test (in the accelerated test) shall be carried out for 3 months or more using the above mentioned products as controls.

6.5.2 In the case of drug products containing a new active ingredient, etc., if applications are being filed for multiple products having the same active ingredient, administration route(s), dosage and administration and efficacy and effectiveness in the same dosage form, with only the contained amount being different, the long-term storage test and the severe test shall be carried out on the product which has been indicated to be the most susceptible to the storage conditions in the preliminary tests.

For the remaining products, in principle, it shall be permissible to substitute the performance of the accelerated test for the long-term storage test in the Standards. In addition, even in the case of different drug forms, as long as the specifications for the excipient, etc., are almost the same, the drugs shall be handled in accordance with the above description.

6.5.3 In the case of application for approval of drug products which are as a result of divided manufacturing, and when the packing materials and packing form covered by the application are the same as the packing materials and packing form for which approval and licensing have already been obtained by the manufacturer of the bulk drug, it shall be permissible to attach to the application the stability test results obtained by this bulk manufacturer.

6.6 With regard to the stability test data, which were formerly stipulated so far to be prepared on the bases of the results of test performed by the applicant himself, such data as prepared by partners of the joint development and public institutions or the like (officially designed testing institutions etc.) shall be accepted as application documents if they meet the requirements stipulated under the Endorsement Regulations of the Pharmaceutical Affairs Law.

References:

(1) Yakuzaigaku *42*, 118 (1982)
(2) Woolfe, Drug Development Communication, *1*, 185 (1974–1975)
(3) Carstensen, J.T., J. Pharm. Sci., *65*, 311 (1976)

VI. Proposed FDA Guideline for Stability Testing

R. C. Shultz, Division of Neuropharmacological Drug Products,
Center for Drugs and Biologics, FDA

1. Introduction

The guideline for stability studies for drugs, promulgated in the Center for Drugs and Biologics of the United States Food and Drug Administration, is not a document of mandates which will be enforced in a court of law. It does contain procedures and recommendations that the Administration, based upon its experience over the years in reviewing new drug applications, has found will provide a means for obtaining adequate responses to the requirements of the United States Food, Drug and Cosmetic Act, with regard to drug product stability expiration dating. By following the guideline recommendations, and/or embracing its principles, an applicant can expedite the approval and marketing of new drugs.

The new drug rewrite finalized by announcement in the *Federal Register* of February 22, 1985, and the soon to be announced investigational new drug (IND) rewrite, direct more reliance on guidelines to help the pharmaceutical industry meet the requirements of the Food, Drug and Cosmetic Act, and regulations as they pertain to the marketing of new drugs. The Center for Drugs and Biologics has prepared a series of guidelines in the areas of chemistry and manufacturing controls. One of these is the Guideline for Stability Studies for Human Drugs and Biologics, which will be talked about today.

"The Guideline does not tell an applicant what he *must* do, nor how he *must* go about obtaining stability data, rather, it is intended to provide guidance for the design of stability studies to establish the capacity of a new drug to remain within the specifications which were built into it at the time of manufacture to assure its identity, strength, quality and purity."

To place the Guideline in its proper perspective, a few words need to be said about its gradual evolution to its present stage.

The Stability Study Guideline, first drafted in the 1970s, was prepared by the Stability Guideline Committee composed primarily of volunteers from the New Drug Application review staff of chemists and microbiologists. The charge was to prepare instructions that would identify acceptable information which applications should contain to fully comply with the requirements of the new drug law. The objective was to speed the review process and to bring consistency to the reviewer's decisions throughout the reviewing divisions.

This early document was confined to new drugs introduced to the market place through the full IND-NDA process. It was not finalized, however, before a decision was made to expand the Guidelines's coverage to include drugs introduced through abbreviated new drug applications and, still later, through the product license application procedure for biological products. When the NDA and IND rewrites were published in draft on October 19, 1982, and June 9, 1983, respectively, the Guideline was completely reappraised and adjusted to avoid inconsistancies with the proposals in the rewrite documents. After receiving approval at the Center level, the resultant Draft Guideline for Stability Studies is the one announced in the *Federal Register* of May 7, 1984, as being available for a comment period of three months, which was extended to four months at the request of several segments of the pharmaceutical industry.

Reponses were received from seven individuals, and 48 pharmaceutical manufacturers, each containing multiple comments directed to all but six of the 68 sections listed in the Guideline's table of contents.

Obviously, the careful consideration fully due these hundreds of comments presented the committee with no small task!

The responses were distributed randomly, about five to each member of the committee who agreed to review all of the comments from his assigned respondants in preparation for subsequent discussion by the full committee. The final Guideline, which will be made available by *Federal Register* announcement, incorporates the recommendations and comments in those sections of the Guideline where the committee agreed an adjustment should be made.

2. Drug substance

The reviewing chemist's first contact with a new drug is through the description of the unformulated, biologically active chemical compound in Phase I of an IND. If there is no IND, as for generic drugs introduced so the market through an abbreviated new drug application, references to publications or other documents that may be on file with the Agency, describing the stability characteristics of the unformulated drug substance, may be acceptable *if* the article also includes details of the storage stations, analytical methodology, and methods used to interpret and support its conclusions. A decision must be made by the reviewer, however, that the information concerning the stability of the drug substance, from whatever source, is adequate to meet the requirements of the Act.

The Guideline reflects our belief that these studies made to establish the stability characteristics of the unformulated drug substance is a good time to start to accumulate information about appropriate analytical methodology, and about storage stations for use in dosage form stability studies. The drug substance to be used for obtaining this stability profile, should be a purified chemical compound whose conformation and functional group characteristics can be exactly delineated. This drug substance stability profile is *NOT* a new recommendation made only in our Guideline, thereby calling for additional work to be done by applicants. On the contrary, both the IND rewrite and the NDA rewrite already require such information to be a part of the applications's description of the physical, chemical, and/or biological characteristics of the drug substance:

- *FEDERAL REGISTER*, Thursday, June 9, 1983.
  (48 FR 26739)
  21 CFR 312.23 (a)(7)(ii):
  ... Stability data are required in all phases of the IND to demonstrate that the new drug substance and drug product are within acceptable chemical and physical limits for the planned duration of the proposed clinical investigation.

  21 CFR 312.23 (a)(7)(iv)(a):
  A description of the drug substance, including its physical, chemical, and/or biological characteristics... and information sufficient to support stability of the drug substance during the toxicological studies and the planned clinical studies.

- *FEDERAL REGISTER*, Friday, February 22, 1985.
  (50 FR 7494) 21 CFR 314.50 (d)(1)(i):

DRUG SUBSTANCE: A full description of the drug substance including its physical and chemical characteristics and stability, and such specifications and analytical methods as are necessary to assure the identity, strength, quality, and purity of the drug substance; that is, specifications relating to stability, sterility, particle size and crystalline form.

With this information on hand, changes in the conformation and functional group characteristics of the unformulated drug substance should already have been identified as well as the storage station effecting the change, be it by heat, light or humidity. Since the primary objective of this early study of the unformulated drug substance is to *detect* changes in its physicochemical properties, storage under stressed conditions, preferably unprotected by enclosure in a container, when applicable, is suggested. Chromatographic methods, such as thin layer chromatography and/or high performance liquid chromatography in several solvent systems are usually adequate for detection. Such a study need be conducted only once for each new drug substance produced by the same manufacturing process. For the purpose of our Guideline, these are short term studies to identify labile functions only. Similar studies may be useful to the manufacturer, however, for application to other lots for the reevaluation of bulk drugs.

Should changes occur in any of these characteristics, then further efforts should be made to specifically identify and measure the extent of the molecular alteration which accounts for the change. Stability indicating, quantitative analytical methodology to measure these structural and chemical properties must be developed in order to do so. The method should be validated for accuracy, precision, sensitivity and specificity.

To complete the bulk drug substance profile, it is well to include studies in solution where the chemical reaction kinetics of any degradation can be most accurately determined, and where the pH of the solution may prove to be an important factor in its decomposition. Physical changes, such as changes from one polymorph to another polymorph, should also be examined.

Ideally, this drug substance stability profile will be developed along with its characterization as a chemical entity very early, or even prior to the submission of an IND. The earlier the better, since in determining the drug substance stability profile the basic elements needed for a stability study protocol of the drug product will also have been identified.

Many of those responding during the comment period questioned the role of the bulk drug substance stability profile, assuming that the drug substance might always be required to bear an expiration date. An expiration date is required only for antibiotic drug substances.

There is little question that the benefits returned to the pharmaceutical manufacturer during a drug product's lifetime, fully justifies the necessary expenditure of time and effort in the design of an acceptable stability study protocol for that product. If after communication by telephone and letter, there remains a need for consultation in the development of the protocol between government scientists in the reviewing division and their industrial counterparts, meetings can be arranged upon request. Once the stability study protocol is approved, it can be applied with confidence that the generated data will be acceptable.

3. Drug product

Each formulation proposed for the dosage fom of the new drug substance to be marketed will have to have its own stability study protocol. For even though the active chemical substance can degrade in only a finite number of ways depending upon its structural and chemical characteristics, the stability study protocols for the drug products will differ depending on the possibility of chemical interaction with excipients and on physical changes associated with the characteristics of the dosage form. For example, one of the properties for which change with time may be difficult to detect in accelerated preliminary studies, is a dissolution rate change for the active ingredient from the drug product matrix of inactive components.

The stability study protocol development is definitely a team effort, utilizing input from the organic chemist, the quality control chemist, the pharmacist and the statistician, both while it is in the hands of the drug developer and the drug application reviewer. FDA's statisticians, for example, are called upon to confirm not only that the stability study describes a design that is suitable for statistical evaluation, but also that statistical methods are used in the sampling and testing procedures, and in analyzing the data.

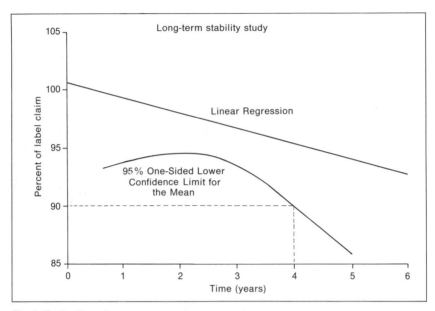

Fig. 1: Evaluation of an expiration dating period

3.1 Statistical evaluation of an expiration dating period

One acceptable approach for inclusion in a stability study protocol is given as follows in our guideline:

If a drug characteristic under study might be expected to *decrease* with time, the time should be determined at which the 95% one-sided lower confidence limit for the mean degradation curve intersects the lower acceptable specification limit. For example, in the figure 1 an expiration dating period of four years would be granted. If an *increase* is to be analyzed, an upper limit on a degradation product for example, the 95% one-sided upper confidence limit for the mean would be used. In other cases, the drug characteristics may have both an upper and lower specification limit creating a special case where the two-sided 95% confidence limits for the means would be appropriate.

Using this approach will assure, with 95% confidence, that the average drug characteristic of the batch is within specification up to the end of the expiration dating period. Statisticians conferring on this approach might well agree on a more appropriate alternative, if it is offered in a proposed stability study protocol.

Extrapolation of an expiration period beyond the range of storage times actually observed, is dependent upon an assumption that the degradation relationship must continue to apply through the estimated period and this may not be valid. For this reason, an extrapolation should always be verified by actual stability data as soon as these data become available.

Our statisticians, writing further in the guideline, make additional recommend-ations concerning the content of the stability study protocol as follows:

3.2 Design Considerations for Long-Term Studies Under Ambient Conditions:

3.2.1 Selection of the batches

A stability study is intended to establish, on the basis of testing a limited number of batches of a drug, an expiration dating period applicable to all future batches of the drug manufactured under similar circumstances. This approach assumes that inferences drawn from this small group of tested batches extends to all future batches. Tested batches must, therefore, be representative in all respects of the population of all production batches of that drug and must conform with all quality specifications.

Ideally, the batches selected for stability studies should constitute a random sample from the population of production batches already produced. In practice, the batches tested to establish the expiration dating period are usually the first clinical study batches produced, and there is a possibility that future changes in the production process will result in the obsolescence of the initital stability study conclusions. For this reason, additional batches should be subjected to stability studies whenever a substantial change occurs in the manufacturing process or formulation.

3.2.2 Number of batches

A sufficient sample of the batches should be taken to adequately assess, within batch and between batch, variability and to test the hypothesis that a single expiration dating period for all batches is justifiable. At least three batches, and prefereably more, should be tested to allow for some estimate of batch to batch variability. The recommendation of three batches is a compromise between statistical and economic considerations.

3.2.3 Selection of samples

Container-Closure and Drug Product Sampling Considerations:

Selection of drug products from the batches chosen for inclusion in the stability study should be carried out in such a manner as to insure that the samples chosen are representative of the batch as a whole; that is, they should be sampled randomly. Sampling of at least two containers for each sampling time is encouraged.

In deciding how to sample the individual dosage units for assaying, consideration should be given to the possible variability associated with the product. As a rule, the sampling of dosage units from a given container should be done randomly, with each dosage unit having an equal chance to be included in the sample. In the case of large containers, it may be suspected that dosage units near the cap of a bottle may have different stability properties than dosage units located in other parts of the container. In this case, it may be desirable to sample dosage units from all parts of the container suspected of giving different stability results. For dosage units sampled in this fashion, the location within the container from which they were taken shoud be identified. This information should be included when presenting the results.

3.2.4 Testing sequence

Sampling Time Considerations:

The sample times should be chosen so that degradation can be adequately characterized, i. e., at sufficient frequency to determine with reasonable assurance the nature of the degradation curve. Usually, the relationship can be adequately represented by a linear, quadratic, or cubic function on an arithmetic or a logarithmic scale.

The degradation curve is estimated most precisely, in terms of the width of the confidence intervals about the estimated curve, around the average of the sampling times included in the study. For this reason, sampling more frequently around the end of the desired expiration dating period is encouraged, since this will increase the average sampling time toward the desired expiration dating period.

The stability study protocol for each new drug need not be in a separate submission requiring approval separate from the NDA as a whole. Our Guideline lists considerations which have been found to be generally acceptable for the design of characteristics for specific dosage forms to be evaluated during stability studies in addition to the labile functional groups of the drug substance. The items of concern, which have been found to change in some cases with storage time, are not intended to be mandatory requirements. They are only suggested factors which we believe are of universal concern and characteristically associated with that specific dosage form and they may, or may not, be of concern to each individual manufacturer of every drug in that dosage form. An applicant, of course, may choose to follow alternative procedures either with or without prior discussion with FDA, though discussion is recommended in the interest of avoiding unproductive effort.

In any case, the approved stability study protocol is nothing more than the detailed plan described in an approved NDA which has been applied to generate and analyze acceptable stability data in support of the expiration dating period. This same protocol, or plan, may also be followed to provide additional stability information to support an extension of the dating period. The protocol gaining approval would be in accordance with the Guideline recommendations, where applicable.

The studies of the dosage form in its market container will, of necessity, have to be conducted first on samples which are only representative of production lots, since they are usually manufactured on a smaller scale for clinical studies of product efficacy. The Guideline defines such data as primary stability data and indicates that it is acceptable in a NDA only when accompanied by a commitment to confirm the expiration period, which was granted on the basis of storage data from those clinical samples, by completing similar studies with production scale lots after approval of the application.

We prefer, and so indicate throughout the Guideline, that the first three lots of the drug manufactured for distribution in the market place be used for this confirmation. The only exception to this "first three" recomendation is that any production lots ot meeting marketing specifications, which have been approved in the NDA, are not to be included in the count. We believe that the use of the first three marketable lots for this confirmation of the expiration date, will avoid inadvertent bias in the selection of lots to be reported to FDA. Where multiple size products of similar concentrations are involved, alternatives to the "first three lots" recommendation may be acceptable on a case by case basis.

Although generally agreeing with some comments that only the smallest and the largest container-closure size need be studied for stability, provided that any intermediate size have identical compostion, the committee listed as exeptions to this general rule all sizes of multiple unit containers such as aerosols and parenterals, where it is recommended that all sizes be studied. Exceptions may be granted for some parenteral formulations if supported by adequate justification, especially where the drug substance stability profile shows it to be stable in solution.

The Guideline recommends that chromatography be included as an analytical method at each test interval, in all dosage form stability study protocols.

New peaks appearing in the chromatograms with time, could mean the introduction of degradation products or of leachables from the container-closure combination. Efforts will be expected to be made by the drugs manufacturer to identify and determine the pharmacological properties of the degradation products, particularly their toxicity. The reviewers who must have access to the full composition of the container and closure, may make proposals for the identification of leachables depending upon the magnitude and significance of the contamination.

The Guideline continues to recommend tests at frequent intervals to confirm that the sterility of Small Volume Parenterals and Large Volume Parenterals is maintained during storage studies. This may be done by a variety of means, as stated in the Guideline. Suitability tests of the container-closure integrity may be insufficient if the integrity does not continue to be maintained during storage due to changes in the physical characteristics of the system.

It is required for drugs marketed through the NDA and product license procedures that lots used for stability testing comply with all approved specifications for the product in its market package. Expiration data generated from drug product's falling short of this requirement in any respect will be used for support of an expiration dating to the fullest extent possible and should be submitted.

Our new drug application reviewers would like to be informed about any stability testing conducted during the product development stage. Whether they were stability studies of exploratory formulations, or of the drug in packaging later rejected. The information gives the reviewer added confidence to support a conclusion that a rational, scientific process was followed during the development of a new drug in a stable composition.

After the drug application has been approved, the acceptable stability study protocol should be followed for the generation of additional data from the first three marketable production lots to confirm the expiration dating period granted on the basis of clinical samples.

For drug products formulated from drug substances showing little tendency to degrade under stressed conditions, stability testing may be performed at three-month intervals during the first year, six-month intervals during the second, and yearly, thereafter. This protocol is also needed in assessing changes made through supplemental applications.

For example, a supplement that proposes a change in the formulation of the drug product, in the supplier of the drug substance, or a change in the container-closure system, will require new stability data from a study of the altered product to confirm that there is no significant stability change during storage up to the previously approved shelf-life. Stress storage data, submitted in tabular form for convenient comparison with the original data obtained under similar conditions, may provide sufficient support to permit continued use of the previously approved expiration dating period, but is should be accompanied by a commitment to obtain confirming data under the storage conditions stated on the product label. A similar commitment to conduct confirmatory stability testing is usually all that is required for the interchangeability of adequately standardized polyethylene containers, a new manufacturing facility, the use of reprocessed materials which otherwise meets specifications, or a new container fabricator if in compliance with the NDA commitments made by the previously approved fabricators.

For biological products marketed through the Product License Approval route, the stability study recommendations in the Guideline are very much like those to be followed for the NDA route. If the applicant's biological products development section had been adequately represented when the stability study protocols were established, that protocol should be followed for product license changes made for the marketed product. These are similar to the NDA supplements but are called amendments to a Product License application.

The Stability Guideline concludes by summarizing general recommendations concerning the content of stability proposals. By checking your submissions against this five point outline before you mail them, many of the reviewer's requests for additional information will be avoited.

It is suggested that stability reports include the following information and data to facilitate decisions concerning the stability proposals:

4. General Product Information:

4.1 Name of drug and drug product or a biological product.
4.2 Dosage form and strength.

4.3 Labeling and formulation. (The application should provide a table of specific formulations under study when more than one formulation has been studied.)

4.4 Composition, type, and size of container-closure.

5. Specifications and Test Methodology Information:

5.1 Physical, chemical, and microbiological characteristics and prior submission specifications (or specific references to NDA or USP/NF).

5.2 Test methodology used (or specific reference to NDA, prior submissions, or USP) for each sample tested.

5.3 Information on accuracy, precision, and suitability of the methodology (cited by reference to appropriate sections).

5.4 For biological products, a description of the potency test(s) for measuring biological activity, including specifications for potency determination.

6. Study Design and Study Conditions:

6.1   Description of the sampling plan, including:

6.1.1 Batches and number selected.

6.1.2 Containers and number selected.

6.1.3 Number of dosage units selected and whether tests were conducted on individual units, or composites of individual units.

6.1.4 Sampling times.

6.1.5 Testing of drug or biological products for reconstitution at the time of dispensing (as directed on the labeling), as well as after they are reconstituted.

6.2   Expected duration of the study.

6.3   Conditions of storage of the product under study (temperature, humidity, light).

7. Stability Data/Information:

7.1 Lot number (research, pilot, production) and associated manufacturing date.

7.2 For antibiotic dosage forms, the age of the bulk, acitve drug substance(s) used in manufacturing the lot.

7.3 Analytical data and source of each data point, e.g., lot, container, composite, etc. Pooled estimates may be submitted if individual data points are provided.

7.4 Relevant information on previous formulations or container-closure systems should be included (or referenced, if previously submitted).

8. Data Analysis and Conclusions:

8.1 Documentation of appropriate statistical methods and formulae used in the analysis.

8.2 Evaluation of data, including calculations, statistical analysis, plots, or graphics.

8.3 Results of statistical tests used in arriving at microbiological potency estimates.

8.4 Proposed expiration dating period and its justification.

8.5 Release specifications (establishment of acceptable minimum potency at the time of initial release for full expiration dating period to be warranted).

In conclusion, I would like to present the names of the present Stability Guideline Task Force responsible for the Stability Study Guideline and who have agreed to remain together as a standing committee to keep the Guideline up-to-date in its recommendations.

Stability Guideline Task Group Members:

Edward A. Fitzgerald
Donald E. Hill
Bernard P. Goldstein
Ernest G. Pappas
Donald J. Schuirmann
Kenneth Furnkranz
Raja Velagapudi
C. T. Viswanathan
Leonard A. Ford
G. Poochikian
M. Theodorakis
Robert C. Shultz, Chairmann

VII. State of the official regulations concerning stability testing of pharmaceutical products in the EEC

Huyghe, B., Mees R., Brüssel

1. Official Regulations concerning Stability Testing of Belgium

Belgium was the very first country to issue well-defined standards through an initiative taken by the Medicines Commission who, at the time, published guidelines on stability tests that had to be included in the registration file.

Specific requirements with regard to the stability of medicines were laid down in Belgium in the context of the Medicines Act of 25 March 1964 and more specifically of the implementing legislation regarding the manufacture and marketing authorization of drugs. Article 20, 8° of the Royal Decree of 6 June 1960 states that the holders of a licence to manufacture, prepare or import medicinal products shall be obliged, when the stability of a medicinal product has not been proved beyond doubt, to guarantee the stability of the product within the limits of the expiry date which they mention on the label.

2. General Introduction

The shelf life must be assessed on the basis of stability tests.

Of course, the pharmaceutical industry cannot, for obvious reasons, wait for the medicines to reach their expiry date under normal circumstances and, moreover, no medicinal product, be it either in solid or in liquid form, can keep its properties for an indefinite period of time.

The microbiological, physico-chemical or synthetic-chemical (= polymerization or condensation), and chemical (such as oxidation, hydrolysis of esters or amides, or else racemization, decarboxylation or depolymerization) effects on drugs are well known to all. Yet, in abstract studies these reactions occur separately while in reality this is not always the case. In fact, it is often found that several of these reactions occur simultaneously and that they are affected differently by environmental conditions.

This amounts to saying that the degradation process is extremely complex; it is not surprising, therefore, that the EEC Directives leave manufacturers ample opportunity to study the problem in depth.

Now that the provisions introduced by Directive 75/318/EEC relating to analytical, pharmacotoxicological and clinical standards and protocols in respect of the testing of proprietary medicinal products have been in force for some ten years, we find that there are large discrepancies in the standards that various EEC Member States require or "do not require".

Using a survey of the current situation in the various EEC countries, it is intended to demonstrate that, in spite of the differences in the protocols of the specific stability tests, it would be possible, given a minimum of goodwill and common sense, to establish guidelines that are common to all stability testing programmes and to standardize them so as to obtain, at least for the general criteria, well-defined requirements applicable to all stability tests.

As the only objective of the stability tests is to guarantee the therapeutic efficacy and the innocuity of a proprietary medicinal product in the course of the distribution process, these guarantees should be concerned with:

● the active ingredient content;
● the absence or the limitation of degradation products;
● galenical conformity tests, especially when these can affect tolerance and the intensity of the therapeutic response.

That is why every registration dossier must/should include the stability data on both

● the *raw materials used,* and
● on the *specialized form* in which it will be marketed (in a commercial packaging).

3. What can be said in 1985 about the Raw Materials?

Although all the Member States did require stability tests on the finished product right away, this was not the case for stability tests on the raw materials and it has taken some countries some time to require them; even now, stability tests on the starting materials are not yet compulsory in some countries.

Of course, in the case of known starting materials references to publications in this area should suffice, but when choosing well-tested batches account will have to be taken of changes that may take place in the physical structure of the active principles (density, specific surface, crystallographic system) as well as of the degree of purity when passing from the experimental stage to industrial production, as indeed considerable changes occur when scaling up the production of starting materials, which may seriously affect the stability of the drugs.

4. What can be said in 1985 about Medicinal Products in Pharmaceutical Form?

It would be ideal for the pharmaceutical companies if they could simply wait for medicines to come to the normal end of their shelf-life. Obviously, this is impossible for economic reasons; hence medicines are subjected to accelerated testing.

Although EEC Directives provide general guidelines for running stability tests, some provisions laid down by national laws or regulations are more restrictive than others.

Thus, national approaches already differ:

4.1 Acceptability of accelerated testing

- *Federal Republic of Germany* does not generally accept it ("nicht anerkannt");
- *Denmark* does not accept it;
- *France* is very reluctant to accept it because, although accelerated testing is authorized, the period of stability is determined taking account *solely of real-time tests*;
- *U.K.* accepts it... but only as a support;
- *Italy* accepts it *for novel molecules only* and requires it to be completed by data on the stability under ambient conditions as and when they become available;
- *Ireland* accepts it *on condition that* it be accompanied, by results of tests under ambient conditions performed over a period of 1 to 2 years;
- the *Netherlands* accept it in principle at the start of the tests; *Luxembourg and Belgium* accept it; their requirements are included in the decisions taken in the standards and protocols of the former joint Benelux Drug Registration Service.

4.2 Number of batches required to perform the stability tests

It may be said that divergencies are very small indeed:

- *Federal Republic of Germany* requires a minimum of 2 batches
- *Belgium* and *Luxembourg* require at least 2 batches;
- *Denmark* still requires 3 batches;
- *France* does not determine the number of batches but requires at least one;
- *Greece*: the number of batches varies; no minimum is specified;
- *Ireland* requires at least 3 batches;
- *Italy* stipulates "several batches", usually 3;
- the *Netherlands* require a minimum of 2 batches;
- *Spain* and *Portugal* require at least 1 batch.

It is clear from the preceding that most countries require *at least 2 batches*, which amounts to saying that, in practice, most often 3 are required, thus joining those who have put their minimum at three.

It would be fairly easy to harmonize the requirements of the EEC Member States in this area: indeed, bringing the required number of batches to three would raise few, if any, objections. Anyhow, the quality of the drugs would greatly benefit from it.

4.3 Number of temperatures required in stability tests

- *Federal Republic of Germany* requires tests in real time to be carried out not only at ambient temperature (to be specified in the dossier) but also at 4 different temperatures;
- *Belgium* does not require a fixed number of temperatures; it may be freely determined by the manufacturer but usually results should be given at least three significantly different temperatures.
  As the decomposition of the active principles at the high temperatures used in the tests is often different from that at ordinary temperatures, there is a tendency to adopt a modest temperature not exceeding 45 °C. The proposed temperatures sould include the observations made on samples kept at the suggested storage temperature;
- *France* has no official acceptable temperature limits, but three fixed temperatures used in accelerated stability tests are usually chosen from among the following ranges:

  from $+25\,°C$ to $+30\,°C$
  $\quad\;\;\; +30\,°C$ to $+40\,°C$
  $\quad\;\;\; +40\,°C$ to $+45\,°C$
  $\quad\;\;\; +50\,°C$ to $+55\,°C$.

  The $+25\,°C - +30\,°C$ range, which is slightly superior to the average temperature of a temperature zone, may be used as a reference for the values obtained at the ambient temperature of that region;
- *U. K.* requires three significantly different storage temperatures, one of them being the ambient temperature, but it prefers the use of temperatures below 45 °C, which makes it possible in some cases to avoid errors of interpretation;
- *Greece:* as was the case with the number of batches to be used the choice of temperatures is left at the manufacturer's discretion;
- *Ireland* accepts 50 °C as the maximum temperature and requires one of the temperatures to be the ambient temperature;
- *Italy* at present still leaves the choice of temperature at the discretion of the manufacturers;
- *Luxembourg* and the *Netherlands* requie three significantly different temperatures.

From the various national positions regarding both the acceptance of accelerated testing and the number and choice of temperatures to be used in trials, it may be concluded that:

- the large majority of EEC countries does not reject the use of accelerated tests;

- most countries require that the trials include tests under ambient conditions;
- in respect of the temperatures, two main requirements appear in all countries:
  - the almost compulsory inclusion of the ambient temperature among the chosen temperatures, as it is this temperature which affects the normal degradation of the medicinal product during the whole of its shelf-life;
  - the preference for the use of fairly moderate temperatures not exceeding 45 °C in accelerated stability tests in order to avoid errors of interpretation that may occur as a result of the fact that the decomposition of the active principles at high temperatures often differs from the decomposition at ordinary temperatures.

4.4 Desirability to require stability tests in a high humidity atmosphere and/or in the presence of sufficient light

It would be highly desirable to require stability tests in these conditions, when the drug, because of its composition or mode of packaging, proves to be sensitive to the effect of these factors.

At present, two European countries – the Federal Republic of Germany and the U.K. systematically provide for controlled humidity conditions.

The three *Benelux countries* require them when they find that the drag is sensitive to it.

France will shortly require that the behaviour of drugs should be examined under conditions of excessive humidity, i.e. a relative humidity between 80 and 90 per cent, generally associated with a temperature between 30° and 45 °C.

Italy requires ambient conditions and humidity.

As a matter of fact, both humidity and light are two factors which will gain in importance in the future. Until a few months ago all the Member States of the EEC – except Italy – were situated in the temperate climate zone with an annual mean temperature of about 15 °C and a relatively high atmospheric humidity of about 60 per cent. This is no longer so now. In addition to Italy, Greece, Spain and Portugal also have a Mediterranean or subtropical climate with annual temperatures averaging 15 °C–22 °C and with a humidity that differs from that of the temperate zone.

5. Conclusions

From this overview of the existing situations in the EEC Member States it can be *concluded* that, in spite of the remaining differences, a common view on many a problem already exists or is in the making, which opens up fresh avenues for concerted action.

For example, it is agreed unanimously that:

- the stability tests be carried out on drugs in their commercial package;

- the specificity of the evaluation method used should be demonstrated so that impurities and the degradation products can be detected;
- the degradation products must, as far as possible, be identified, their toxicity be studied and their acceptable rate be defined;
- the physical stability of the product must always be part of the stability studies. Of course, in this respect the requirement will depend on and will vary according to the galenical form of the medicinal product;
- the expiry date be CLEARLY indicated on the inner and outer package. (All the EEC Member States require the month and the year, except Ireland which, in addition, requires the day);
- as far as the active ingredient content of a medicinal product (generally set at 90–110% of the indicated dose in most of the EEC Member States with the exception of Belgium which requires 95–105%) is concerned, one may wonder if Belgium has not been the forerunner of the requirement inserted in part 1 (E) (2) of Council Directive 75/318/EEC of 20 May 1975 by Council Directive 83/570/EEC of 26 October 1983 (in force at the 1st of November 1985) which reads as follows:

    "Unless there is appropriate justification, the maximum acceptable deviation in the active-ingredient content of the finished product shall not exceed ± 5% at the time of manufacture.

    On the basis of the stability tests, the manufacturer must propose and justify maximum acceptable deviations in the active-ingredient content of the finished product up to the end of the proposed shelf-life."

Finally it is believed that it ought to be possible to harmonize the various national standpoints.

If we take a common denominator of the different views, we can finally reach greater uniformity in the way the stability tests are conducted by advocating for example:

- the acceptance of the principle of accelerated testing in all EEC Member States. These tests must be carried out on the drugs as they are presented in their final package or, at least, in a package that offers the same protection from factors or agents affecting the shelf-life of the drugs;
- the obligation that one of the tests be conducted under ambient conditions over at least a 1 to 2-year period. (Indeed, applicants have a fairly long period of time at their disposal, if only because of prolonged clinical experiments when the tests were organized with foresight at the outset);
- that the number of temperatures that may be required for the tests be restricted to a minimum of three, one of them at ambient temperature and the highest at 45 °C or 50 °C at the most, on the understanding that these three temperatures be sufficiently apart for Arrhenius' law to be applied;
- that calculations and results determining the period of stability on the basis of an extrapolation of the velocity constants observed at higher temperatures be mentioned in detail in the dossier.

The primary task of the Working Group on the Quality of Medicines, set up by the Committee for Proprietary Medicinal Products, is to secure a uniform interpretation of the provisions of the EEC directives relating to the quality of medicines.

It is up to this working group to consider whether the provisions regarding the stability tests are sufficiently clear or whether they should be supplemented by a note for guidance addressed to the pharmaceutical industry and the competent authorities.

VIII. Requirements of the Licensing Authority of the Federal Republic of Germany concerning the Stability Testing of Drug Products, with special reference to Phytopharmaceuticals

F. W. Hefendehl, Institut für Arzneimittel des Bundesgesundheitsamtes, Berlin

1. Stability Tests according to the draft of a Drug Testing Guideline, Section dealing with Quality

In § 26 of the German Drug Law of 1976 (AMG), the Federal Minister for Youth, Family Affairs and Health is obliged to set out general administrative instructions covering the requirements the Federal Health Office (BGA) has to place on the analytical, pharmacological-toxicological and clinical data to be submitted with an application for licensing a drug product (1).

The section of these administrative instructions, called Drug Testing Guidelines, dealing with quality so far only exists in draft form. The requirements contained therein are based strictly on those of the corresponding guidelines of the European Economic Community (EEC) (2).

To establish the stability of a drug product, the draft of the Drug Testing Guideline, Section on Quality requires the following: The experiments on stability must be described in such a way that they enable the shelf life proposed by the applicant to be deduced. If the possibility exists that harmful degradation products may form from a drug product, then details must be given of the method for their estimation and of the upper limit of content accepted. In all instances where there is any conceivable risk of interaction between the drug and its container and especially in cases of injectable preparations or aerosols for inhalation, a description of such interaction must be provided. It must be possible to draw a conclusion from the analytical results concerning the duration of stability and the need for any protective measures during storage.

The other statements in the draft concern special provisions or exemptions which will be discussed later, during consideration of stability tests of drugs with plant constituents (Phytopharmaceuticals).

2. General Requirements of Stability Tests

At first sight, the requirements of the Licensing Authority concerning stability tests appear rather sparse. This discrepancy is explained when one looks at the basic definition of stability in the APV Guidelines "Stability and Stability Testing of Drugs" (3): "Stability means the maintenance of the quality defined in the drug product specification until the end of the manufacturer's stated shelf life." Thus the requirements of stability tests arise out of the specifications for the finished product, which must be fulfilled throughout the proposed duration of stability. In certain cases, shelf life specifications might also appear in addition to those for the finished product. The former might be extended a little further if the quality of the finished drug is thereby not fundamentally influenced.

Just a few of the important basic requirements of stability tests will now be considered.

2.1 Number of Batches to be tested

The investigations of stability must be carried out on at least 2 batches of the finished drug product in the packaging proposed for marketing. This figure of 2 batches represents a compromise between statistical necessity and economic considerations. In fact, values from only 2 batches are below the limit from a statistical point of view, as for example is shown in a special supplement to "The Gold Sheet" of May 1984 (4). The pharmaceutical manufacturer must be aware that 2 test batches are only adequate provided they show no major deviations from each other.

2.2 Duration of Testing

The duration required of the stability tests is directly related to the stability claimed. In view of the forthcoming obligatory clearly stated expiry date, the following applies: Up to a proposed stability of 3 years, the half-time rule is applicable, i.e. the results, for example, of a long term test of 18 months duration can establish, provided the results justify it, a stability of 3 years. The storage conditions used must correspond to those proposed for the marketed product. Experiments under stress conditions can only be used to confirm the results of long term tests. In the case of new drug substances, stability tests on the substance itself can provide further supportive evidence. If a stability of over 3 years is claimed, then stability must be tested over the entire shelf life by appropriate experiments under the storage conditions proposed for the marketed product.

2.3 Equivalence of Tests that were carried out under other Conditions

If the stability tests were undertaken in a container, the material specifications of which did not correspond to the final container, then the equivalence of the two packaging materials must be established, with particular reference to the permeability to moisture and light.

If the composition of the test batches differs from that of the finished product, the results – with appropriate explanatory justification – can then be accepted if it represents a multiple or a fraction of the final composition, or the content of active ingredient deviates only slightly from this and the composition of the excipients is practically constant. Additional tests of the physical parameters of the finished product may be necessary.

2.4 Testing Frequency

As a minimum requirement, results of an initial and a final test must be submitted. However in general this is only sufficient in the case of relatively stable drug products. Results from intermediate investigations are generally needed to enable a clear trend to be detected.

2.5 Test Parameters

These originate, as has already been said, from the various specifications of the final product. It is important that those physical parameters that are relevant to stability are also adequately tested, in addition to the external characteristics, the content, the test for degradation products and the limit for harmful breakdown products. All specifications should, wherever possible, be tested by objective methods – for example – the colour of solutions on the basis of Pharmacopoeial instructions (5).

2.6 Stability Specificity

The methods used in the stability tests for measuring content must be suitable for quantitatively detecting the characteristic structural and chemical properties of each active constituent and differentiating the latter from degradation products. The methods must only determine the actual content of the active ingredient. Even relatively non-selective techniques fulfill this requirement provided breakdown products can be separated beforehand with adequate certainty, or their absence is firmly established – here information is required of the sensitivity of the method. Although it is theoretically possible to quantify the breakdown products and then calculate the content of active ingredient, in practice this is generally difficult to achieve.

2.7 Stability Overages

Stability overages as a means of compensating for loss of potency during storage are permitted up to a maximum of 10%, provided this is not done to prolong the stability period beyond 3 years (6).

In exceptional cases, this limit of 10% may be exceeded with periods of stability up to 3 years. The need for stability overages must be based on the results of the stability tests.

3. Foreign Documentation and Responsibility of the Pharmaceutical Manufacturer

Documents from other countries will be accepted by the BGA provided they completely fulfill the above-mentioned requirements and are submitted in German or English. It is noticeable that these requirements concerning stability tests are in some areas less stringent than the corresponding ones in the APV Guidelines. This is because the draft of the Drug Testing Guidelines, Section dealing with Quality, is closely based on the requirements of the EEC. Furthermore, it should be borne in mind that official requirements are not of such a nature that they interfere with the

4. Stability Tests of Phytopharmaceuticals

4.1 Definition

In the following discussion, phytopharmaceuticals will be regarded as drug products whose active constituents are crude drugs or preparations of crude drugs. Pure substances isolated from plants or highly concentrated mixtures of active constituents from crude drugs will not be considered here.

4.2 Peculiarities of Crude Drugs and Crude Drug Preparations

A crude drug or a crude drug preparation is considered in its entirety as an active constituent. Thus the discussion about the division of all the constituents of a crude drug into active components, coeffectors and indifferent substances loses a little of its importance. Quality, even of a crude drug where the activity-determining substances are well established, is not solely determined by their quantitative determination. These active substances must be viewed and evaluated in association with the other components that make up the complete crude drug. Under these conditions, crude drugs in which the active substances are as yet only inadequately identified – if at all – but whose effectiveness can be demonstrated, may also be included in the group of medically usable crude drugs.

Nevertheless, one must regard the view that a crude drug or crude drug preparation as a whole represents the effective constituent, as a temporary expedient, which can only apply until further scientific investigations of and with therapeutically used crude drugs provide other standards. This necessity arises from the fact that no absolute identity of substances can be expected from plant to plant or even from batch to batch, certainly not under the conditions of the normal worldwide crude drugs market of today. The possibility of avoiding or limiting this disadvantage through the cultivation of genetically uniform plant material has so far only been achieved in a few cases.

The tests for quality assurance and for reproducibility of a given quality must take account of these realities. All available steps must be taken to ensure within the acknowledged range of natural variations, that the most homogeneous material possible is selected. Only in this way can the assertion that phytopharmaceuticals also represent drugs whose reproducible quality enables a consistent therapeutic effect to be expected be upheld.

4.3 Stability Tests of Crude Drugs and Crude Drug Preparations

On purely practical reasons, the discussion of the problems in stability tests of crude drugs and crude drug preparations is divided into a consideration of those with known active substances and those in which the active substances have not yet been identified. No distinction is however made between drugs of strong and weak activity, since from the standpoint of quality, both must be treated exactly the same. Even a crude drug or its preparation with low potency, usually taken for longer periods, must always show a consistent quality if it wishes to justify the claim of being a reliable drug. The correlation: weakly active – more limited testing, is, for a drug, not acceptable.

As has already been stated concerning definitions: A crude drug or crude drug preparation is regarded in its entirety as an effective constituent in which individual substances or substance mixtures can be present which are counted as activity-determining substances. The individual members of such a mixture are described as components.

4.3.1 Single Crude Drugs and Crude Drug Preparations with Known Active Substances

With crude drugs one can assume that the activity-determining principle consists of a mixture of components. These components may belong to a single group, e. g. ethereal oils or two or more groups e. g. ethereal oils and flavonoids. The investigations of stability must establish that the total amount of the components of one group varies only within the specification i.e. does not fall below 90% of the theoretical value or a minimum amount established by a pharmacopoeia. At the same time, it must be demonstrated, e. g. through chromatographic techniques, that the component mixture within the active group of substances does not alter greatly. Intentionally, no fixed limit is given here, because the decision is an individual one for each case, based on the reasons given by the applicant. The degradation of a minor component in an ethereal oil clearly has a different effect on a drug than the cleavage of a glycoside into the respective aglycone and sugar. Nevertheless, every transformation or degradation of individual components of the substance group should be evaluated to see whether significant instabilities of the crude drug or of its preparation can result. It is important that the documentation gives exact details of the tests and that copies of chromatograms, spectra etc are submitted. The reference parameters are the results of the initial tests on the batch concerned. Changes in the substance should not only be considered from a chemical point of view, but also in terms of the therapeutic effect which, for example, could lead to different pharmacokinetic relationships. An aglycone obviously has completely different properties that the respective glycoside.

As with drug products of a chemically synthetic nature, it is not the job of the regulatory authorities to prescribe what methods are to be used. These are to be chosen by the pharmaceutical manufacturer as appropriate for each task. The costliest method does not always provide the most useful results. A well produced and properly evaluated thin layer chromatogram can often enable better predictions of stability than high performance liquid chromatography. As was said at the beginning, in relation to the general problems of specificity of stability tests, special care must be taken with multicomponent mixtures to ensure that breakdown products, even with chromatographic techniques providing a high degree of separation, really can be differentiated from the components that are present at the start of storage. In addition to the tests mentioned here for qualitatively and quantitatively constant composition of the active substances (which can differ from the tests of chemically synthetic substances only through the complexity of the component mixture), with phytopharmaceuticals, the constancy of the other components of crude drugs and crude drug preparations must also be monitored. It is obvious that this test can in no way detect to total amounts of all substances, but must be global in character. So, for example, it is possible to make observations or statements by the chromatography of different polar fractions of the crude drugs or their preparations. The relevance of changes in the composition is to be assessed and also viewed in connection with changes in physicochemical parameters such as solubility, appearance, pH value etc.

4.3.2 Single Crude Drugs or Crude Drug Preparations, whose Active Substances are not known

The stability testing of crude drugs and crude drug preparations where the active substances have not been identified has to be limited to determining and evaluating the overall composition of the crude drug. In this case, it is necessary to show groups of constituents of different polarity by separate chromatography. The fingerprints so obtained have to serve as the basis for evaluation. The assessment of the qualitative and quantitative behaviour of reference substances alone is generally not adequate for a stability prediction, since these substances were chosen more or less at random from the many plant constituents. The predictive usefulness of their stability behaviour can however be increased if substances are selected that are known to be labile. Admittedly this type of stability test is somewhat less than satisfactory. The licence applicant of such products is accordingly required to opt for the shortest possible shelf life. A more reliable basis for evaluation would be obtained if biological tests were to be used, appropriate to the indications claimed, in addition to chemical, physicochemical and physical methods. Unfortunately, research in this area has so far not progressed very far.

4.3.3 Crude Drug Mixtures or Mixed Crude Drug Preparations with Known Active Substances.

There are no major differences compared to the single crude drugs or crude drug preparations. Difficulties arise however because the number of substance groups and individual components to be evaluated increase. With mixtures of several or more crude drugs, this can lead to the situation where only limited predictions are possible. Identical substance groups from 2 or more crude drugs could be treated together, i. e. the ethereal oil content of the oils of several crude drugs can be determined and specified at the same time; the composition of total mixture is to be correspondingly checked. This type of test is naturally then only permissible if the type of activity of the components justifies it – i. e. if the glycosides of 2 or more plants, for example, show identical therapeutic effects.

If this is not the case, then the contents of the individual crude drugs must be separately evaluated, which if necessary can also be carried out by a stability test of the individual crude drugs or their preparations. This will be considered again later.

The other stability tests are the same as those for single crude drugs.

Analytical problems with mixtures of crude drugs or crude drug preparations can, in many cases, be avoided if one keeps the number of active constituents as low as possible. It seems highly questionable whether there are still good reasons for having mixtures of more than 6 constituents.

4.3.4 Crude Drugs Mixtures or Mixtures of Crude Drug Preparations with Unknown Active Substances

Stability Tests of mixtures whose active substances have not been identified can (as in the case of single crude drugs) only be undertaken on the basis of fingerprint chromatograms. It must be realised that with increasing numbers of crude drugs, the ability to make stability predictions becomes so low that the analytical effort is no longer worthwile. Here it is possible to take advantage of the permitted exceptions to the rules, which are summarised below.

4.3.5 Quality Assessment of the General Characteristics of Various Dosage Forms of Phytopharmaceuticals during Stability Tests

In essence, there is no difference here between chemically synthetic drug products and phytopharmaceuticals. However it must be pointed out that the evaluation of sensory or organoleptic characteristics assumes great importance, especially in the case of crude drugs and crude drug preparations where the active substances are unknown. Nevertheless, an evaluation of these characteristics requires objective criteria, which if necessary are to be taken from the field of food chemistry (7).

A constant source of discussion are cloudiness and precipitations with liquid preparations. Thoma's view that serious and marked cloudiness is a sign of deficiency in manufacture and that only slight turbidity is acceptable and should be established by appropriate objective criteria is to be supported. A similar opinion is given in the Pharmacopoeia Helvetica, which however only relates to conditions on dispensing. Irrespective of the nature of the change in quality (which is only rarely explained) and therapeutic effect, it is quite unreasonable for the patient to be given an oral solution which is sometimes clear, sometimes cloudy and other times cloudy with a sediment – especially if this cannot be resuspended.

4.3.6 Special Provision for the Stability Testing of Phytopharmaceuticals

The draft of the Drug Testing Guidelines, Section dealing with Quality, contains two special provisions which particularly affect phytopharmaceuticals.

Firstly the stability testing of mixtures of crude drugs or crude drug preparations can be carried out with the individual crude drugs or groups of crude drugs provided two conditions are met.

1. The individual crude drugs or drug preparations must lie in a matrix which corresponds to that of the finished product or is very similar.

2. Proof must be submitted that no interactions are likely between the individual crude drugs or preparations. Whereas the latter point can be relatively easily established with solid preparations, great difficulties can arise with liquids (8).

It is important to point out that this special provision can only be used if it is conclusively shown that the total mixture cannot be analysed with reasonable expense. Examples of "reasonable expense' are: thin layer, column, high performance liquid and gas chromatography, but not gas chromatography coupled with mass spectrometry. Grounds for claiming exemption are also required for the second special provision:

If a qualitative and quantitative quality control of the contents of the drug product cannot be carried out, it is possible to establish quality merely by a suitable examination of the starting materials and a validated manufacturing technique and then to undertake only physical and sensory tests as stability controls. Under these circumstances, stability is to be limited to 1 year.

4.3.7 Summary and outlook

Stability testing of phytopharmaceuticals must demonstrate that the specifications of the finished product are maintained throughout the shelf life. In this respect, phytopharmaceuticals are no different to drug products with chemically synthetic active consituents. The difficulty in assessing stability tests of crude drugs and crude drug preparations arises out of the claim that a crude drug or its preparation is to be regarded in its entirety as an active constituent and is thus to be evaluated as the behaviour of a wealth of different substances. What we are actually dealing with is a drug product that generally consists of several active constituents and a multitude of excipients, some of which at least are involved in the efficacy of the product. Not until more research has been carried out will it be possible to prove to what extent e.g. highly purified extracts – where stability can be more reliably evaluated – can be used instead of the crude drugs or their preparations.

The stability testing of phytopharmaceuticals indeed recognizes a few specific peculiarities such as: Testing for constant composition of active substance mixtures, quantitative overall measurement of inseparable active substances or substance mixtures of several crude drugs and the global testing of the overall composition of a crude drug; separate testing of active constituents or the limiting of stability control to physical and sensory tests in well founded exceptional cases.

When all is said and done however, stability testing must enable a statement to be made as to how long the specifications of the end-process control can be adequately maintained. In this respect, phytopharmaceuticals are treated no differently than drugs with chemically synthetic ingredients. Thus the APV Guidelines "Stability and Stability Testing of Drugs" for example, can be applied almost in their entirety to phytopharmaceuticals, provided some of the above-mentioned peculiarities of this group of therapeutic agents are taken into account. If phytopharmaceuticals are to be regarded as equally valuable as other drugs, then their willing inclusion in a general Stability Guideline is necessary.

References

(1) West German Drugs Law of 24. August 1976. Official Gazette I page 2445 Article 1, Law relating to Medicines (Arzneimittelgesetz)
(2) EEC Guidelines 75/318/EEC, Offical Journal of the European Community L 147/1 of 9 June 1975 and 83/570/EEC, Official Journal of the European Community L 332/1 of 28 November 1983
(3) See for example Pharm. Ind. *47*, 627 (1985)
(4) The Gold Sheet, Special Supplement, May 1984
(5) European Pharmacopoeia Volume I, page 54
(6) See for example, Dtsch. Apoth. Ztg. *120*, 2546 (1980)
(7) G. Harnischfeger and H.G. Menssen in: Qualitätskontrolle von Phytopharmaka (Ed. G. Harnischfeger), Georg Thieme Verlag, Stuttgart, New York, 1985; page 15
(8) A. Moosmayr in: Qualität pflanzlicher Arzneimittel (Ed. G. Hanke), Wissenschaftliche Verlagsgesellschaft mbH, Stuttgart, 1984; page 136.

IX. Stability Testing of Pharmaceutical Products: Official State Requirements in France: Analytical Approach and Schema for the Study of the Stability

by F. Pellerin, D. Baylocq and N. Chanon Centre d'Etudes Pharmaceutiques, Université Paris Sud

1. Introduction

The stability of a drug depends on its retaining the activity and safety which it was designed to possess. This is a short definition, but the evaluation of stability involves many aspects which require very varied tests and the relevant regulations developped in various countries worldwide are fairly varied also. This means that the pharmaceutical industry is obliged to carry out research in a variety of fields: kinetic, mathematical and chemical tests, studies of the compatibility of the constituants amongs themselves, and even with the containers. There are also studies of the self life under very varied climatic conditions and the fixing of expiry dates. All these parameters constitute aspects of the stability study; the specific investigation of each yields an accumulation of overlapping data and, in the end, means very high financial costs when tests have to be adapted or new ones devised to satisfy the requirements of the regulation.

A stability study may appear to be a particular section of the drug registration dossier, involving the confirmation of a certain number of legal criteria or criteria established by common practice together with studies conducted under a variety of conditions to determine the stability of the drug in various climatic zones. Such an approach, which is necessary in principle, should be taken into consideration in the study programme. However, it rapidly becomes apparent that it is insufficient to evelute the behaviour of the drug and can even be the source of erroneous interpretation.

A more realistic modality consists of establishing the stability data from all of the physical and chemical data acquired over the development of the drug from the raw material to the finished product. With this approach, the stability is seen to be a consequence of the properties of the drug, it is derived from the study of the chemical reactivity of the molecule and the transformations which it undergoes under various conditions or under the action of reagents or auxiliary substances which will be added to the pharmaceutical form.

It is on the basis of these data, assembled in an explanatory dossier, that the stability of the active drug and the pharmaceutical products in which it is contained can be evaluated. Such an approach is able to predict and elucidate the mechanisms of degradation, establish methods of investigation, justify their choice and fix the limits of detection. The legal requirements can be satisfied on the basis of this knowledge.

On the basis of this attitude, an analytic approach and a study schema ensuring conformity with legal requirements are presented, by proposing successively, illustrated by several examples, the establishment of the stability programme, the choice of techniques and, thirdly, the modalities of studies of the shelf-life and interpretation of the results in the context of the legal requirements.

The aim of this lecture is not to review and discuss each topic of official text in order to establish a list of requirements but to formulate a number of concepts to explain the modalities of stability studies, to describe the study techiques capable of guaranteeing the safety of a drug for the whole of its shelf-life.

2. Stability – Study Schedule

Maintenance of the efficacy and safety of the drug is the verification of its pharmaceutical quality, its therapeutic activity and the absence of microbiological, toxicological or biological changes implies the participation of all drug specialists at all stages of development and, notably, of analysts and pharmacists.

2.1 During the development stage, the pilot manufacturing process is concentrated around problems of formulation and the compatibility of the constituents amongst each other as well as verification of technological criteria during tests carried out under accelerated or hostile conditions. In this way, a considerable amount of data is amassed which serves as a basis in the elaboration of the industrial manufacturing process. At this stage, changes of type or degree may emerge which demand the modification of the formulation and of the stability parameters to be tested.

2.2 The Role of the Analytical chemist

Official texts show that the analytical chemist plays a crucial role in several areas (1) (2).
– Participation at all stages of the progress of the drug; the analytical chemist remains the centre of all stability studies, since his presence is required whenever qualitative or quantitative determination is necessary, and various areas of analytic specialisation are involved: chemical, physical, biological, enzymo-immunological, etc.
– Fundamental studies of the behaviour, reactivity and degradation of the drug and, at the same time, the selection and validation of analytical methods.

– Establishment, monitoring and execution of programmes, if necessary in liaison with specialists in mathematical or statistical studies.
– Monitoring of the storage conditions, studies of leaching and interactions with packaging materials.
– Stability studies under various conditions.

The data obtained make it possible to resolve the various problems which arise:
– The conditions of storage, transport, use, the compiling of technical data sheets and of leaflelts intended for practitioners (doctors and pharmacists) and users.

Finally, the evaluation of stability goes beyond the areas of efficacy and safety; it demands as variety of studies, including those concerning shelf-life and storage conditions, as well as the establishment of an expiry date, which is simply the culmination of these studies.

2.3 In order to attain this objective, many parameters must be determined,

● Technological parameters: manufacturing criteria;
● Physical and physio-chemical: solubility, crystallinity;
● Chemical: Reactivity, tests for, identification or detection of degradation products;
● Tests of the finished product: conversions, reactions, incompatibilities.

These tests are carried out under a variety of conditions. This yields an impressive list of parameters to be determined and checked which is likely to dishearten even the most enthusiastic researchers and the best organised units, as well as to stretch financial resources, and this has led many registration departments to draw up a checklist of the parameters required ... as well as those which are added in order to avoid the risk of rejection or questioning by the governing authority. The problem must be approached realistically.

In the opinion of the authors, this realism depends principally on certain general facts: stability is established on the basis of data acquired progressively and included in the pharmaceutic file. Quite apart from the regulations, the compilation of a detailed dossier of this type can help to save time. If we consider that the development of a drug may extend over 8 to 10 years, then this file includes all the pharmaceutical studies and is not seen as the static state at a given moment, but rather a dynamic report expressing the development of the product and its stability.

In addition, the logical and realistic study of stability following a well-structured programme – which is clearly described for the registration authorities – avoids the drawbacks of the checklist system, which indicates an impressive succession of parameters to be checked and may result in the carrying out of pointless studies. Each speciality constitutes a separate entity and demands an appropriate specific study. If the stability study is restricted to the verification of a checklist of this type, it may give a false sense of security when in fact the investigation or verification of some essential criteria may not be included.

This is a mechanized approach – to avoid the term "robotized" – and the intellectual passivity which it involves may seriously impair the real knowleldge obtained of the stability.

The stability evaluation programme should not be drawn up in order to comply with all the items of the regulations but, rather, should adapt itself to them. The regulations and, in particular, the European Directive and Notice to Manufacturers express only general concepts, which each manufacturer must adapt as necessary. We consider that the success of a stability study should not be assessed in terms of whether it responds to and satisfies all the official headings. A stability study should be the outcome of reflection in each particular case and of a free and justifiable choice of the criteria to be adopted and the tests to be carried out. Compliance with official requirements will result from a study conducted in this way.

This is one of the reasons for the stress we have put on several occasions on the importance of the approach to stability studies (3) and of compiling an effective file presenting the data necessary for a scientific explanation of the pharmaceutical file. In the same way, in France the European Directive has given rise to a Notice to Manufacturers, which was published by the authorities and has recently appeared in a French periodical (2). This same journal is soon to publish an explanation and a description of an example in order to provide manufacturers with the features necessary to draw up their own files and also a study outline which will provide them with an effective guide.

3. Setting up the Study

The evaluation of the stability of a drug involves two successive phases: experimental tests of the raw materials and of the finished product, followed by interpretation of the results and their application to the progress of the drug.

3.1 Investigation of the active principle: Purity and reactivity

During development, the analytical chemist must take care to define the characteristics of the product which must be retained throughout its development and to identify the mechanisms of degradation, in order to reduce their extent, determine the extent of degradation and, if necessary find chemical or physical methods or additives (preservatives, antioxidants...) for slowing or limiting this process. It is on the basis of the data obtained that the stability and storage conditions will be determined and, eventually, the duration of storage fixed. Without going into the details of all the verifications carried out, we well develop in particular certain topics which must be investigated: purity, reactivity, external factors, knowledge of which controls stability and constitutes the basis of the formulation of the drug as well as its progress and its behaviour under various conditions.

The purity of a raw material intended for pharmaceutical use is, obviously, a criterion which does not require much development. The presence of an impurity may have a negative effect not only in virtue of its toxicity, but also because of possible catalytic effects, such as those often encountered with inorganic impurities. Conversely, in the case of equilibrium reactions, the presence of a degradation product – if it is not involved in either toxicity or activity – restricts the shift in equilibrium (5).

3.1.1 Reactivity of the molecule

The principle route of approach to stability, or to the constancy of a raw material, lies in the exploration of its physicochemical properties or, in other words, of its reactivity. This study is the precedent to establishing specifications, such as those involved in the study of the half-life and metabolism. These concepts of the reactivity and the importance of the physico chemical properties of the functional groups which we have frequently stressed (6) have been taken up again in the Notice to Manufacturers. This is also true of the changes undergone by organic compounds during forced degradation reactions. We consider them to be the very basis of stability studies and will demonstrate this by means of examples.

Kinetics of chemical reactions. The study of chemical kinetics has an important place in the study of stability, as in biopharmacological or drug-metabolism studies. The role of chemical kinetics will not be developed here. The accelerated study of the stability of drugs and pharmaceutical preparations is based on the application of fundamental principles and theories of physical chemistry and chemical kinetics. It is based on Arrhenius' equation $K = Ae - \Delta H_a/RT$ where A is a constant related to the entropy of the reaction and ΔH_a is the heat of activation. *Whenever the relation at high temperature (T) is linear, it is feasible to study the prediction of stability storage temperatures.* The application of the laws of physical chemistry and kinetics, the subject of GARRET's work in this field is now well known in the pharmaceutical industry. The interpretation of the stability of a chemical drug, and the forecasting of its shelf-life, generally rest on a study of the active constituent in aqueous solution at high temperature; this is followed by the variation of the physicochemical properties such as the development of the infra-red absorption spectrum, and, very often in the ultra-violet, that of an electrochemical property measured by the development of an intensity/potential curve or by the appearance of a breakdown product detected by chromatography.

It is not always sufficient to measure a property and its variations; the difficulty lies in knowing the development of the reaction and the nature of the products formed. The concentration of the active component by a spectral method does not always yield information on the stability, since the transformation may affect only a part of the molecule and the product formed often has spectral characteristics little different from those of the original component. *The stability is determined by the concentration of breakdown products, assuming that* the component does not itself undergo another reaction. Whenever several linear or convergent reactions develop, the relation between the kinetics at various temperatures and the shelf-life becomes illusory. The result of a physical measurement such as absorbance is uninterpretable: it represents globally the results of reactions for which the kinetics are different. Here again, knowledge of the reactivity and the transformations should precede kinetic studies.

Finally, studies under various conditions and the application of kinetic methods lead to a considerable number of data that are often hard to interpret. The reactivity of the functional groups will often allow a simplification and especially to explain the stability of the drug.

3.1.2 General study procedures

A knowledge of the stability can be approached through the study of reactions conducted under various conditions, dry or in solution: the effect of temperature (37°−45 °C) or of light in acid or alkaline media, or of oxidizing or reducing agents. The experimental transformation reveals *the weak points* of the molecule and facilitates the identification and determination of the structure of the components so formed. The results obtained by relatively aggressive means, direct the search for these same products after conservation of the finished product under conditions of use. They also allow chemically tolerable limits to the breakdown products to be fixed, before the toxicological problem is addressed. At the same time, the experimental transformation justifies the methodology of the study.

The primordial importance of reactivity in predicting stability, identifying degradation products and selecting methods of investigation is illustrated by the following examples.

3.1.2.1 Reactivity in solution: Role of the solvent

The study of the reactivity should include tests in solution. The importance and the role of the solvent are well known to the analyst who exploits its properties for analytical purposes. The solvent intervenes through its power of dissolution and its involvement in chemical proton-exchange or redox reactions. The use of photometry or oxide-reductometry made by the analyst is well known in the study of different solvents. These reactions in solution are also applicable to the study of the stability of the molecule, and it should not be forgotten that numerous liquid or semi-liquid pharmaceutical formulations enclose organic solvents that are far from being inert; polyethylene glycol, glycol, polysorbates, for example, change the pH of the solutions and have an effect on the reactions of the molecules. In suspensions or emulsions, the partition of the chemical component between these two phases affects the reactivity; the partition coefficient is therefore one of the measures of stability.

3.1.2.2 Reactions of cyclisation are common; glutamic acid can be cycled by heating in aqueous solution aa pyrrolidon-carboxylic acid. The breakdown of aspartam is

also an example of a cyclic reaction that is well known in food chemistry; a derivative known as diketopipetazinic is formed. The stability, like the purity, of this sweetener is not only linked to its content of cyclic derivatives; the breakdown ends, in effect, with the hydrolysis of the ester and amide groups, leading to phenylalanine and aspartic acid.

3.1.2.3 Equilibrium reactions between the dissolved molecules and their breakdown products constitute essentially a factor of stability. In aqueous solution, an equilibrium reaction is established between sodium noramidopyrine methane sulphonate (NAMS Na) and methylaminoantipyrine (MAA). Solutions kept away from light and air remain stable.

The extraction of MAA by chloroform to determine its concentration (7) immediately displaces the equilibrium. Also, the breakdown of NAMS Na follows two different routes: hydrolytic, according to (8) or oxidative, according to (9). In any case, the breakdown leads to the formation of methylaminoantipyrine (MAA) with or without yellowing due to methylrubazonic acid. Gas-phase chromatography or thin-layer chromatography or liquid-phase chromatography (7) allow the formation of these products to be followed and the stability to be monitored. The presence of MAA in pharmaceutical formulations in small proportions (1 to 2%) maintains the equilibrium. Amino-4 antipyrine is only present in traces, not exceeding 0.05 percent; its increase would correspond to a displacement of the equilibrium in the medium under the influence of an external factor (dilution, air, light).

3.1.2.4 Chelation reactions.

Chemical chelation reactions are a cause of instability of organic molecules, going as far as to cause the disappearance of therapeutic properties. They are most often envisaged from the standpoint of protecting the stability, through the addition of a component or a chelator, in a medical form, such as tetracemate which masks the traces of metallic cations and suppresses their catalytic action. The formation of a chelate between a metal and the drug is often the cause of a breakdown or of the instability of the molecule; this leads, as in the case of gentamycine or polymyxine (10), to the diminution, or even the suppression, of therapeutic activity. This fact should not be forgotten. Any time an organic molecule offers two functional groups capable of linking with a metal to form a 5- or 6-sided ring, chelation should be envisaged because of the new properties it might confer on the molecule: chelation takes place in the presence of traces of the calcium, magnesium or zinc salts in the excipients. It can also be shown that such a reaction does not bring about the formation of a soluble chelate.

The formation of metal chelates often affects the excipients, a good many of which are applied elsewhere, for analytical purposes, as chelating agents. The possibility of these reactions should not be neglected when drug formulations are being prepared. For example, bismuth salts, with sorbitol or other polyols (11), form a chelate of known structure, water-soluble in an acidic medium (12). The reaction is based on insoluble bismuth salts (as nitrate, carbonate) in aqueous liquid media incorporating, in suspension or in solution, flavouring excipients or additives and ingredients of certain foodstuffs and drinks: lactic or citric acids; metaphosphates, polyols, etc. (13) (14).

Other factors

Two other factors are also an integral part of the investigation of stability: Radiation and temperature.

3.1.2.5 Role of radiations

The primordial role of light radiations merits attention, since they result in very diverse reactions. The photo-transformation of 3-pheny-2-butanone oxime goes as follows, with the formation of nitrile (15):

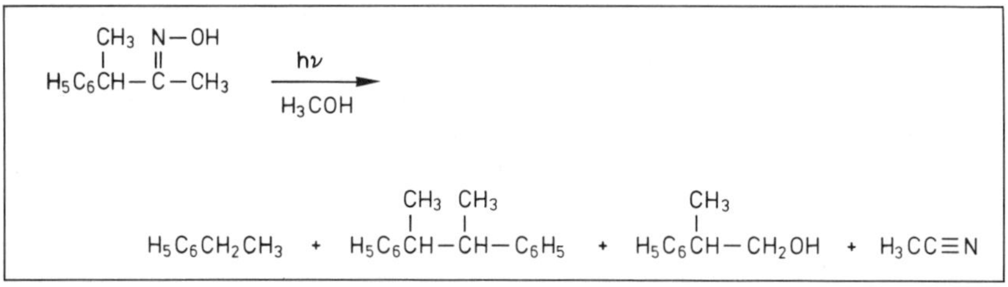

Fig. 1: Photochemical degradation of 3-phenyl-2 butanone oxime

The photolysis of pentobarbitol causes the rupture of the pyrimidine ring, according to BARTON (16).

The photo-oxidation of phenothiazine, with the formation of N- and S-oxides, is well known and has been particularly studied by HEYES and SALMOM in the case of fluphenazine and its esters (17).

The importance of photochemical reactions implies the necessity of determining the stability, under the influence of light, of all organic drugs, by determining the reaction mechanisms and the nature of the products formed. Another consequence of the photosensitivity of drug molecules is research on protective materials. The choice of containers and packaging is particularly important especially in the case of plastics which are themselves sensitive to light radiation or sterilizing radiations. This study is essential throughout the development phase of the drug.

Sterilization by gamma rays is sometimes the cause of breakdown in packaging or medical/surgical equipment. It cause the modification of the mechanical and technological properties of the materials (solidity, colour, elasticity, etc.) and the products formed can be the cause of migration. Such is the breakdown of PVC

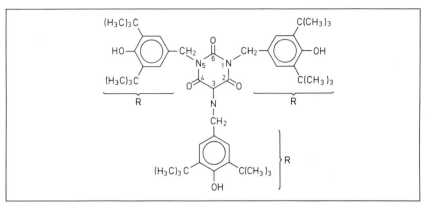

Fig. 2:Decomposition products of goodrite 3114 caused by Gamma rays
1. Tris-(di-tert-butyl-3,5 hydroxy-4-benzyl)isocyanurate

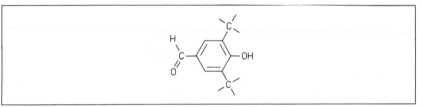

2. Di-tert butyl-3,5 hydroxy-4-benzaldehyde

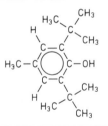

Fig. 3: Decomposition products of
1. B.H.T., Di-tert-butyl-3,5-hydroxy-4-toluene caused by Gamma rays

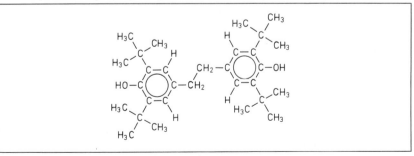

2. Bis-(di-tert-butyl-3,5-hydroxy-4-toluene)

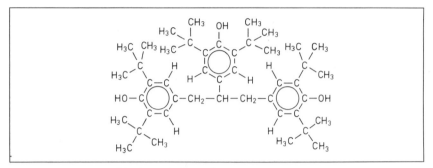

3. Tris-(di-tert-butyl-3,5-hydroxy-4-toluene)

followed by DTA (18). Sterilization by radiation can also affect additives in materials such as antioxidants. With C. Majcherczyck (19) (20), we have shown, for example, that GOODRITE 3114 is broken down by Gamma rays; at first, hydroxyl groups are oxidized to form quinones; then the molecule is split to yield an isocyanurate and finally an aldehyde, the nature and structure of which have been determined by mass spectrometry. In the case of BHT, the same procedures (HPLC, MS) have demonstrated the formation of the dimer.

These examples demonstrate the importance of the following factors for the pharmaceutical industry:

- the need for constant composition of plastic packaging materials:
- the false sense of security which can result from the acceptance of interchangeable additives on the pretext that they are included on a positive list;
- the need to include studies of leaching between container and contents in stability studies of the packaged drug. Any change in the composition of the packaging necessitates further stability studies. Finally, an "undertaking by the suppliers of the container" guaranteeing that he will adhere to the composition and report any changes made, is necessary for packaging materials as for the raw materials.

3.1.2.6 Role of temperature

The part played by temperature in stability studies is obvious and is included in all regulations. In general, "Studies of forced degradation" imply storage at high temperature under various conditions of humidity (21). (table 1)

In fact, there is some degree or ambiguity; the tests at various temperatures correspond to several objectives. In other words, the pharmaceutical laboratory has to organise its studies at different temperatures in such a way as to obtain results which yield a maximum of conclusions. These studies should take the following points into account: to active principle

Table 1: Abstract from Notice to applicants EEC, Sept. 1985
Part II F: Stability

---

1. Proposed shelf life (depending on the type of container and storage precautions). When necessary the shelf life after reconstitution of the product or when the container is opened for the first time.

2. Information concerning stability, including physical stability, of the finished product:
   - Number of batches tested
   - Storage conditions
   - Methods employed
   - Description of containers
   - Analytical methods (if different to those in Part II E) and specifications
   - Results of tests and interpretation

3. Stability tests on active constituent(s)
   - Number of batches tested
   - Storage conditions
   - Methods employed
   - Description of containers
   - Analytical methods
   - Results of tests and interpretation

4. Validation of the methods employed

- temperature is a way of accelerating a reaction;
- it makes it possible to predict degradation processes, to quantify and identify or detect degradation products and consequently to validate the method used in the stability study;
- the result of forced degradation make it possible to define in a second step the conditions of storage and the alterations of both the active principle and the pharmaceutical formulation to undergo deterioration;
  the results of forced degradation is not the objective of to fix an expiry date but only yield a first approximation, which is then confirmed by means of a study in real time at normal room temperature.

3.2 Pharmaceutical Dosage Form Stability Test

The Notice to Manufacturers gives very concise indications concerning the carrying out of tests on the pharmaceutical form.

These are based on the results obtained on the chemical reactivity of the active principle and its degradation process.

They must be conducted according to a protocol adapted to known characteristics of the active principle as well as to dosage form features.

These tests aim at bringing out degradation products that may appear in the dosage form and thus suggest optimal storage conditions (with or without any special protection against heat, cold, humidiy or light).

They should be carried out on at least three batches.

The study takes into consideration the following aspects:

- Organoleptic features
- Physical characteristics particular to the dosage form (tablets, suspension, injectabilia) and main quality parameters in function of the form
- Monitoring the active principle
- Assessment of content in degradation product
- Developing the appropriate methods.
- Degradation products interaction between excipient and active principle and, generally, between the components
- Product-container interaction
- Limit test for preservative, additives, antioxydants, etc...

Once more we are faced by an imposing list of parameters to be checked. Here too the reactivity and functional organic analysis data will provide a valuable contribution, as a few examples will demonstrate

3.2.1 Moisture

The reactivity of organic components is not limited to solution phenomena; it deals also with reactions that occur in the absence of solutions or in dry preparations. In fact, it cannot be asserted that the reaction occurs in the absence of solvent. The manufacture of pharmaceutical formulations may involve the use of solvents that are evaporated during drying; also, certain excipients retain not insignificant amounts of water (up to 20% in the case of starch). This "hidden" water in the constituants may become liberated during manufacture, causing, as a result of liquefaction or humidification, the reaction of the components present.

Thus, as was shown above, certain pharmaceutical excipients, such as polysorbates, hydrogenated oils, polyoxyethylene glycole and, in a general way, the excipients in all ointment formulations have considerable dissolving power; the dissolution of the components in the medium causes the reaction to start. Their dissolving power is even the cause of incompatibility with the plastic materials and significant exchanges between the recipient and its contents (22).

3.2.2 Antioxidants

The effectiveness of the additives needed to maintain stability by blocking reactions or degradation is related to their often marked reactivity and to that of other components present. The study of chemical transformations is essential to avoid errors or the use of poorly active or even sometimes useless substances. Sodium

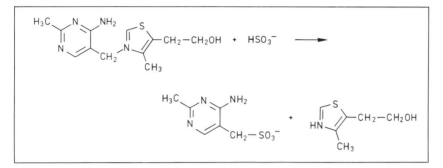

Fig. 4: The breakdown of thiamine by sodium-bi-sulphite

bisulphite protects ascorbic acid from oxidation; in contrast, the breakdown of thiamine by sodium bi-sulphite restricts the use of this antioxidant (23).

It is not sufficient to show that oxidation has occurred and to identify the mechanism of the reaction. The choise of an antioxidant depends on the equilibrium potential between the redox mechanisms of the oxidizable compound and the antioxidant (24). The optimum concentration of the antioxidant – not to be confused with upper limit allowed by law – the synergism of mixtures of antioxidants, their consumption during shortage, and the minimum concentration required to ensure its effectiveness up to the end of the product's shelf-life, are determined by reactivity studies which justify and guarantee effectiveness.

3.2.3 Functional group analysis and prediction of stability

The methods of functional group analysis can be applied to the determination of drug stability. The reaction of ascorbic acid on amino-acids fixes their concentration under various conditions. The presence of these two types of compounds may be the cause of incompatibilities in the colouring of drugs. This fact was observed with C. Majcherczyck (25) and made it possible to determine the reaction mechanism and to produce a diagram analogous to that for the reaction between amino-acids and ninhydrin. Ascorbic acid is oxidized to dehydroascorbic acid in the lactone form. The determination of amino-acid liberated from the ammonia and finally a duplication of the molecule is obtained. The compound has been isolated and its structure determined by NMR and IR spectrometry.

The sjgnal from the carbon atom carrying the side chain of the ascorbic acid is straightened out (72.9 ppm and 75.6 ppm) relative to that observed in the spectrum of ascorbic acid (74.9 ppm).

The displacements of carbon atoms 5 and 6 are identical, but the corresponding peaks are very broad; this indicates a steric constraint reducing the free rotation of the side chain $CHOH - CH_2OH$ and confirms the envisaged structure.

The IR spectrophotometric analysis of the compound shows:

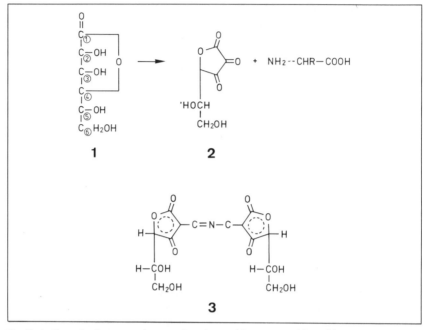

Fig. 5: Action of primary amines and amino acids on ascorbic acid

1. Ascorbic acid   2. Dehydroascorbic acid   3. Reaction product

– a band at $1740 \, m^{-1}$ characterizing the vibration of the $C = O$ valency bond characteristic of unsaturated γ-lactones.
– a wide band at $1500-1700 \, cm^{-1}$ corresponding to the absorption of the vibrations of the deformation of double bonds $C = P \, C = N \, C = C$.
– a band at $1180-1200 \, cm^{-1}$ characteristic of the deformations of the C-O and C-N groups.
– a band at $1500-1700 \, cm^{-1}$ confirms the presence of antimine $(C = N)$ group that is too much surrounded by other atoms to be detectable by the NMR of C_{13}.

3.2.4 Forced Oxidation

The laboratory oxidation of organic compounds by hydrogen peroxide is a convenient means of studying stability and predicting breakdown.

The study of the mild oxidation of sulphamides has been carried out with a view to determining the exact structure of the oxidation products using spectroscopic analytical techniques, and the kinetics of oxidation. The objective of this is to transpose this study to pharmaceutical products to be put on sale, and to study their stability. Four sulphamides – sulphanilamide, sulphamethoxazole, sulphadoxine and probenecide – were oxidized by 20% hydrogen peroxide in 0.5 N sulphuric acid at room temperature under light. The products were separated in a silicone column then purified and crystallized (26) (27).

The method of study used to define the structure of the products is based on:

- Elemental analysis
- UV spectroscopy
- IR spectroscopy
- NMR spectroscopy of 'H and ^{13}C
- Mass spectrometry

The *ultra-violet spectroscopy* is carried out in acidic and alkaline media. Depending on the hypochrome or bathochrome displacements, it allows the appearance or disappearance of NH_2 or OH groups to be followed.

Infra-red spectroscopy in potassium bromide indicates the characteristics of the valency vibration bands and of the deformation of NH_2 and SO_2 groups. The appearance of supplementary bands allows the transformation of the original molecules to be determined.

NMR spectoscopy of 'H or ^{13}C provides information on the environments of the 'H and the ^{13}C as a function of the value of the increments revealed by the chemical displacement read from the spectrum.

Mass spectrometry is carried out by electron bombardment for sufficiently stable oxidation products (azoxy). In the case of more labile oxidation products (diol fraction), chemical ionization with NH_3 gives, with good precision, the molecular weight of the compound.

These procedures allow identification and determination of the structure of the main products, as follows:

Sulphanilamide One diol derivative.   One azoxy derivative (fig. 6)
Sulphamethoxazole Two major products: nitroso and azoxy derivative
Sulphadoxine a nitro derivate

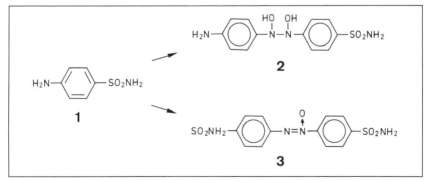

Fig. 6: Oxidative decomposition of sulphanilamide (1) forming one diol-derivative (2) and one azoxy-derivative (3)

The kinetics were determined using HPLC with inverse phase polarity and of zero order.

4. Interpretation of the results and conclusions

4.1 Analytical aspects

Without going into details of the technical techniques employed in the stability study, we do think that it is necessary to mention some specific points.

The tests for degradation products carried out in stability studies make liberal use of chromatographic methods (TLC, HPLC). The procedures adopted require previous validation. It would be erroneous to base any conclusion on a single type of test. The validation of a TLC method involves tests carried out using several different fixed phases and mobile solvents; the selection of the column packing and mobile solvents for HPLC methods is based on several types of studies and optimization of methods.

The validity of a method used to check stability does not necessarily involve the identification of the breakdown product, in some cases it may suffice to demonstrate its presence. This identification may sometimes be very difficult to achieve because it demands the isolation and identification of sufficiently large amounts of these substances. Generally reference substances are not available for use in routine stability tests. In addition, some industries may be unwilling to reveal the nature of the breakdown product for reasons of industrial secrecy. In fact, as long as the detection of the degradation product is based on serious experimental findings which give rise to a reliable test method, the stability method is valid.

It should also be noted that confirmation of stability does not necessarily imply the need to detect all breakdown products... it is impossible to detect the thirty or so substances which may result from the forced degradation of tocopherol under a range of conditions. It is up to each Manufacturer to take a realistic stand and to explain the rationale of the choice made.

We also point out that the EEC directive states that the Expert must express an opinion concerning the stability of the product. According to the definition given by the Société Française de Technique Pharmaceutique, in a stability study the Expert should carry out the necessary experimental verifications (28) and then must give his opinion on the following points:

● the validity of the methods used in controlling stability;
● the chemically acceptable limit values for degradation products at the end of shelf-life, which, if appropriate, should be related to pharmacological and toxicological data;
● the expiry date.

4.2 Technical aspects

The performance of a stability study involves multiple aspects which we have related to the study of the reactivity of the molecule. Another aspect arises from the fact that the national authorities demand specifications which vary from country to country.

In general these specifications are based on the specific climatic conditions in the country but are also governed by custom and habit. It is obviously difficult, if not impossible, to consider every possible case. French requirements are relatively modest, since the "Notice to Manufacturers" gives only a few examples by way of indication (2) (4):

● for ageing tests: three fixed temperatures are usually chosen, from the following ranges:
   $+ 25$ to $+ 30\,°C$
   $+ 30$ to $+ 40\,°C$
   $+ 40$ to $+ 45\,°C$
   $+ 50$ to $+ 55\,°C$
● Special temperatures such as $- 10°$ to $- 20\,°C$
                                $+ 2°$ to $+ 8\,°C$
                                freeze-thaw cycles
● Special conditions: temperature $+ 30°$ to $+ 45\,°C$; humidity 80–90, p. 100

The special conditions correspond to special climatic zones or to products of which the active principle is deteriorated by heat.

The expiry date for use and the acceptance limit for the degradation product at the end of the shelf-life is based on these data. This lower limit is not based on the stability study alone: it also takes into account the toxicological and clinical data as a whole, which demonstrate that at the end of its shelf-life the drug retains its therapeutic activity and that its safety has not been altered.

4.3 Conclusion

The contribution of analytical organic chemistry to the study of drug stability is not limited to the choice and perfecting of the methods most appropriate to each particular case; it also resides in very thorough analytical research into the reactivity of organic molecules. The reactivity explains the transformations, prelude to the prevention of drug breakdown: it is the point of departure for physico-chemical studies of formulation, drug kinetics, forecasts of shelf-life and the fixing of the date of validity. These studies precede the prevention of breakdown by means of appropriate additives and explain the transformation. The requirements on drug stability demand detailed analytical research into the validity of the methods and a solid knowledge of their limitations. These results carry an unquestionable and adequate guarantee of chemical quality and safety of use.

Bibliographie

(1) Notice to applicants EEC III/158/85 EN – Septembre 1985
(2) Directive to manufacturers – S.T.P. Pharma (1985) 1, 734
(3) F. Pellerin et N. Chanon – Sci et Techn. Pharm. (1981) *10*, 341
(4) F. Pellerin et N. Chanon – S.T.P. Pharma (1985) on press
(5) F. Pellerin – Produits et problèmes pharmaceutiques (1967) 22, 16
(6) F. Pellerin – Pure and Appl. chem. (1975) *44*, 579
(7) F. Pellerin et. J.F. Letavernier – Ann. Pharm. Fr. (1973) 31, 3, 161
(8) S. Ono – R. Onishi – K. Kawamura – J. Pharm. Soc. Japan (1966) 86, 11
(9) F. Pechtold – Arzneim. Forsch. (1964) *14*, 258-474-1056
(10) B.A. Newton – J. Gen. Microbio. (1954) 10, 491
(11) L. Vanino – F. Hartl – J. Prakt. Chem. (1960) *74*, 145
(12) F. Pellerin – D. Mancheron – Ann. Pharm. Fr. (1967) 25, 797
(13) F. Pellerin – J.P. Goulle – D. Dumitrescu – Ann. Pharm. Fr. (1977) 35, 281
(14) F. Pellerin – J.P. Goulle – D. Dumitrescu – Bull. Acad. Nat. de Médecine (1976) 160, 268
(15) B.L. Fox – S. Saloman – M. Goldschmidt – Technical report AFML TR 72 – 4 University of Dayton – Janv. 1972
(16) H. Barton – Die Pharmazie (1980) *35*, 3, 155
(17) W.F. Heyes – J.R. Salmon – J. Of Chrom. 194 (1980) 416–420
(18) F. Pellerin – B. Legendre et F. Guillot – Ann. Pharm. Fr. (1982) *40*, 221
(19) C. Majcherczyck – Thèse 3ème Cycle – F. Pellerins' Laboratory – University Paris XI (1985)
(20) D. Baylocq – C. Majcherczyck et F. Pellerin – Talanta (under press)
(21) M. Pesez – Publication de l'O.M.S. WHO – Pharm. 79495
(22) F. Pellerin et D. Baylocq – Labopharma (1983) **31**, 333, 552
(23) Food Tread. Rev. (1976) *46*, 1, 76
(24) F. Pellerin et D. Baylocq – Labopharma (1978) N° 273 p. 130; (1980) N° 340, 535
(25) D. Baylocq – C. Majcherzyck et F. Pellerin – Talanta (1983) *30*, 72
(26) A. de Souza – These Doct. es Sciences Pharmaceutiques – F. Pellerin Laboratory University Paris II (1984)
(27) D. Baylocq – A. de Souza et F. Pellerin (under press)
(28) F. Pellerin – Moderator of an S.F.S.T.P. Commission – S.T.P. Pharma (1985) 1 N° 2

X. Great Britain, The DHSS Medicines Division Requirements

A. G. Stewart, Department of Health and Social Security, G. B.-London

1. Introduction

The licensing of medicinal products intended to be placed on the market of the United Kingdom of Great Britain and Northern Ireland (UK) became mandatory on September 1, 1971, following the publication of the Medicines Act 1968 (1).

The Medicines Division of the Department of Health and Social Security (DHSS) acting as the Licensing Authority (LA) prepared guidelines (2), (3) for industry which included notes on stability testing requirements. When the UK joined the EEC in January 1973, it became necessary to incorporate the requirements of Council Directives 65/65/EEC and, later, 75/318/EEC and 75/319/EEC into the UK guidelines. This was done in subsequent revisions of the UK guidelines. The latest requirements of Council Directive 83/570/EEC and Council Recommendation 83/571/EEC will be included in a fresh revision of the guidelines which is expected to be published early in 1986. This paper mentions the underlying philosophy adopted by the UK Licensing Authority, refers to the training of the pharmaceutical staff who assess the data presented to them, and considers some of the details in the guidelines.

2. The Underlying Philosophy

The UK Licensing Authority does not prescribe the design nor the number or type of tests that need to be performed in stability testing. The system of control of medicinal products in the UK is one of interaction between the pharmaceutical industry, the Licensing Authority and its consultative and advisory bodies – the Medicines Commission, the Committee on Safety of Medicines (CSM), the Committee on the Review of Medicines (CRM), and the Committee on Dental and Surgical Materials (CDSM) with their expert Sub-committees on aspects of pharmacology, toxicology, efficacy, chemistry, pharmacy and adverse reactions. This complex system has considerable benefits both for the industry and for the patient.

The underlying philosophy of such a system of control is that the pharmaceutical industry has the responsibility for the development and marketing of its medicinal products including decisions concerning the appropriate methods of experimental testing prior to trial or marketing. It is considered that the developer is in the best position to know the potential of his drug and that it is his responsibility to pursue each clue presented during testing so that the benefit/risk ratio can be fully evaluated. It is argued that a pre-set programme of studies of defined type and duration may not illuminate problems that may arise as well as the intelligent implementation of a progressive series of short and long-term studies each following up indications given by an earlier one.

The developer, of course, has to defend what he has done and the decisions he has reached to the satisfaction of the Licensing Authority. It follows from this that the Licensing Authority maintains considerable flexibility in reaching a decision. The use of a committee system greatly increases this flexibility. The expert committees that advise the LA are composed mostly of academic scientists with appropriate specialist interest and wideranging international contacts. They are able to base their decisions upon the most recent movement of informed scientific opinion. This flexibility has the advantage that a product can be approved rapidly where the need for its availability is great. It has the disadvantage that the developer cannot plan his programme of experimental testing with the complete confidence that a specified number of successful experiments, which seemed adequate at the time that the programme was started, will appear the same to the consultative and advisory committees viewed against the background of opinion current at the time that the application is considered. The developer, therefore, must keep himself as fully informed as possible by reading appropriate scientific journals and attending symposia such as the International Symposium on Stability Testing.

3. The Pharmaceutical Assessors

The pharmaceutical secretariat in the UK has 27 members of staff from a wide variety of backgrounds and interests. They are grouped together as in the diagram in Annex I. Regional geographical distribution of assessors to companies is done to enable a team of assessors to become familiar with the companies and the personnel in a given region and to deal as consistently as possible with all licensing matters from those companies.

Stability data are required for all new applications for marketing authorisation, for products that are being reviewed by the CRM before the EEC May 1990 deadline; for variations to existing products where appropriate; and for the renewal of licences as required.

Pharmaceutical staff keep themselves up-to-date by attending suitable courses, symposia, seminars and scientific meetings as well as through the reading of scientific journals and periodicals. The staff also have the benefit of direct and informal contact with the members of the expert committees at the monthly meetings and on other occasions. Staff are encouraged to develop a "guideline" approach when assessing each product and to take it on its own merit rather than having a "check-list"

UK DHSS MEDICINES DIVISION
PHARMACEUTICAL SECRETARIAT

ANNEX 1

Head of Branch
Mr. A. G. Stewart (DCPhO)

NE REGION	NW REGION	SE REGION	SW REGION
Dr. J. Purves (SPhO)	Mr. J. L. Turner (SPhO)	Dr. B. R. Matthews (SPhO)	Mr. A. C. Cartwright (SPhO)
Miss S. A. Norton (PPhO)	Mrs. L. H. Davidson (PPhO)	Mr. J. Davenport (PPhO)	Miss D. Hepburn (PPhO)
Dr. A. T. Keene (PhOI)	Mrs. P. M. Clark (PhOI)	Mr. G. R. Ansell (PhOI)	Dr. J. Roe (PhOI)
Mrs. E. A. Baker (PhOI)	Mr. G. Wade (PhOI)	Mr. R. T. Clay (PhOI)	Dr. J. Yeo (PhOI)

BIOLOGICALS	RADIOPHARMACEUTICALS	DENTAL & SURGICAL MATERIALS	NEW CHEMICAL ENTITIES ADVERSE REACTIONS
Mr. J. P. Betts (PPhO)	Mr. A. T. Gray (PPhO)	Dr. M. I. Robertson (PPhO)	Miss R. A. Coulson (PPhO)
Mrs. J. A. Hampton (PhOI)			
Miss B. H. Woollett (PhOI)			

PHYTOPHARMACEUTICALS	MAFF LIAISON AND SUPPORT	INFORMATION/COMPUTER SUPPORT	PARALLEL IMPORTS
Mr. R. L. Smith (PPhO)	Miss M. J. E. Millar (PPhO)	Miss R. J. Smith (PPhO)	Mrs. B. Shersby (PhOI)
	Mr. J. P. O'Brien (PhOI)		

Each Geographical Region has a mix of abridged, varied, renewed and reviewed licence work.

KEY
DCPhO Deputy Chief Pharmaceutical Officer
SPhO   Superintending Pharmaceutical Officer
PPhO   Principal Pharmaceutical Officer
PhOI   Pharmaceutical Officer 1

MAFF   Ministry of Agriculture, Food & Fisheries
       Central Veterinary Laboratories Weybridge.

mentality which can lead to requests for unnecessary data. They are expected to put themselves in the shoes of the different people handling medicinal products by asking, for example, "why test for stability?" and receiving an answer such as "As a *patient* I would wish to have assurance of an elegant medicinal product with a maximum shelf-life, a clear expiry date and of convenient storage. As a *manufacturer*, I would wish to have assurance of optimal quality at a minimum cost knowing that continuing studies would identify areas for product improvement. As a *drug regulatory officer* I would wish to have assurance that the medicinal product presented to the public is what it claims to be and will remain so within its indicated shelf-life under any specified storage condition".

4. The Guidelines

That guidelines are necessary, especially those for stability is shown from a survey made a few years ago in the Department of the questions that were raised in the pharmaceutical assessment of applications for marketing authorisations. Stability testing raised the largest number of questions. As a result the UK guidelines were modified and expanded and appear as Annex 8 in the 1984 HMSO publication entitled "Guidance Notes on Applications for Product Licences" (2).

The whole question of stability is currently under review by the quality working group of the EC Committee on Proprietary Medicinal Products (CPMP). The UK guidelines along with other Member States' guidelines are under consideration. If any here present today know of any difficulties that are being encountered in the evaluation of stability, the CPMP working group will be grateful for your comments and will take due note of them in the revision of the guidelines.

The recent Council Directive (83/570/EEC) and Council Recommendation (83/571/EEC) amend earlier Council Directives some points of which have a bearing on stability.

4.1 Control Tests on the Finished Product (75/318/EEC)

Unless there is appropriate justification, the maximum acceptable deviation in the active ingredient content of the finished product shall not exceed $\pm 5\%$, at the time of manufacture.

On the basis of stability tests the manufacturer must propose and justify maximum acceptable deviations in the active content of the finished product right up to the end of the proposed shelf-life.

In vitro studies on all solid dose forms (including data on the stored product) are required.

4.2 The expiry date must be in plain language (65/65/EEC Article 13.7).

4.3 Pharmaceutical Particulars (65/65/EEC Article 4a.6)

Incompatibilities (major)
Shelf-life, when necessary after reconstitution
   of the product or when the container is opened
   for the first time.
Special precautions for storage
Nature and content of container

   These were required to be implemented by November 1, 1985 at the latest and are being included in the revised UK guidelines.

5. Discussion

5.1 Some effects of Instability

Before going on to consider some of the detail of the UK requirements on stability testing, the reason why medicinal products need to be formulated, manufactured and packaged so as to achieve satisfactory stability might be better understood if some effects of *in*stability are considered:
   These are:

- Loss of active constituent (eg. nitroglycerin tablets)
- Loss of content uniformity (eg. sedimentation impaction of suspensions)
- Increase in active constituent (eg. drying out of gels, evaporation of alcoholic component of solvents)
- Presence of undesirable micro-organisms (eg. in-use contamination of multi-use formulations)
- Production of potentially toxic degradation products (eg. tetracycline)
- Loss of pharmaceutical elegance (eg. colour changes/development of unpleasant odours).

   Turning now to consider the drug substance and then the dosage form.

6. The Drug Substance/Active Constituent

Considerations of stability begin with an evaluation of the active drug substance. Having determined its identity and purity, and with a knowledge of its physico-chemical characteristics the formulator and manufacturer are required to write down its specification and the tests, with limits or criteria of acceptance, which will be applied to meet that specification.
   These may be summarised under the following headings:

- Appearance (colour, odour, texture, crystallinity)
- Identity tests (IR, UV, MP, chemical test)
- Physico-chemical tests (solubility, pH, moisture, loss on drying, particle size, optical rotation, test for polymorphic form)
- Purity tests (chromatography, ash level, heavy metals, trace elements ie those used as catalysts, residual solvents, moisture)
- Impurity profile on manufacture and degradation profile on storage
- Assay (using a method which is sufficiently specific and sensitive to be useful)

Stability testing of the bulk drug substance is against such a specification and is designed to determine the inherent stability characteristics of the molecule.

The UK Licensing Authority requires the following information on new chemical entities, whether for clinical trial or for product licence:

The number of batches examined
The conditions of storage
The analytical methods used
The results obtained (summarised and *discussed*)

The discussion should be in a scientific manner and not merely a reference to tabulated results. The testing should, wherever possible, be carried out on batches of material prepared by the route of synthesis likely to be used for commercial large-scale bulk manufacture. Any particular impurity pattern will thus be accounted for.

These stability testing findings should be reflected in the formulation work on the selected dosage form(s).

7. The Dosage Form

Pre-formulation development studies evaluate the physical and chemical compatibility of the drug substance with a range of excipients and packaging materials. These tests, often limited and accelerated, enable the formulator to decide the most appropriate formulations of the chosen dosage form for the intended purpose. Coupled with data from the stability testing of the drug substance itself on the likely mechanism and kinetics of degradation the formulator is enabled, with the help of his analytical colleagues, to develop stability-specific analytical methods.

To summarise so far,
The stages at which stability testing is necessary are:

- Evaluation of the active drug substance
- During laboratory/pilot scale manufacture of material for clinical trial
- During production scale-up of the final dosage form for marketing
- When any significant variation occurs in the manufacture/specification of the drug substance/dosage form necessitating a request to vary a licence or certificate.

This last point of course, involves any significant change of pack eg. from a glass bottle to a unit dose blister pack.

8. The Heading on Stability

Considering, now, the Annex on Stability in the UK guideline. There are 9 headings:

8.1 Batches examined

The number of batches examined with size and reference should be stated. At least two batches using, where possible, different batches of active constituent are expected to be tested.

8.2 Conditions and duration of storage testing

The time, temperature, humidity and light conditions etc. under which the product was tested should be stated. It must be remembered, when evaluating results, that moisture, oxygen and light, but not temperature, can be controlled by packaging. The choice of fixed, significantly different, temperatures and humidities and/or cycling conditions are left to the applicant's discretion.

8.3 Containers

Details of those used in the test with their closures should be given and where it is proposed to use a different container or closure for marketing, the significance of the differences should be disclosed. Special attention should be given to plastic containers for parenteral solutions where materials added to the plastic in the course of the manufacture of the container may be extracted by the solution under storage test conditions. There is a note in the guideline about any added desiccant or cushioning material.

8.4 Analytical methods

Details are required of the methods used which should be sufficiently specific and sensitive to detect any deterioration that might develop on storage. It must be remembered that official compendial tests designed to detect and identify impurities in the drug substance may not necessarily be suitable for the investigation of degradation products. Council Directive 83/570/EEC now makes it necessary for the competent authorities to inform those responsible for the pharmacopoeia in question when a monograph might be insufficient to ensure the quality of the substance in question.

8.5 Parameters tested

An article on stability testing in the International Journal of Pharmaceutical Technology and Product Manufacture (4) states that the analytical methods used in a well-designed stability test should attempt to cover the four aspects of product stability:

● Chemical
● Physical
● Microbiological
● Toxicological

Physical stability is one area which is often neglected but may be critical where, for example, a change of crystal form or crystal growth in a suspension, cream or ointment could affect the bioavailability of the active drug substance. Another change, that of pH, may affect the stability and consequently the antimicrobial efficacy of the preservative.

With regard to microbiological stability the British Pharmacopoeial test for Efficacy of Antimicrobial Preservative in Pharmaceutical Products is considered to be a suitable test and which may be modified to suit a manufacturer's particular environmental conditions. Modifications and adaptations should be fully discussed under the heading of Development Pharmaceutics. This test gives criteria for the assessment of the preservative efficacy of injections, eye-drops, oral liquids and topical preparations.

8.6 Results

It is helpful to have these expressed in the same way as on the product label, eg. mg/tablet or per 5 ml dose and if subsequent check points can be given as percentage of initial assay, this speeds up evaluation of the data. Where possible, results should be tabulated or presented graphically. A discussion with conclusions should follow the summary of results.

8.7 Proposed shelf-life

This is derived from a consideration of all available data and may be defined as:

"that period for which a product retains the following within specified limits:
– chemical and physical integrity
– resistance to undesirable microbial contamination
– labelled potency
– therapeutic effectiveness
– pharmaceutical elegance"

If only limited data are available, a restricted shelf-life will be given which can be extended in the light of further satisfactory data. The expiry date in plain language was required to be stated on all labels from November 1 of this year.

8.8 Storage conditions, user instructions and Pharmaceutical Precautions

These follow from the discussion of the results and should be given in clear, unambiguous language. Where a product has to be reconstituted or diluted clear directions as to storage after reconstitution or dilution and as to how long it may be safely used is required. Where an injectible solution is to be given on dilution via a parenteral infusion, an indication of compatibility and stability, physical, chemical and biological, with recommended diluents and administration sets, are required.

8.9 On-going Stability Testing

Where a minimum of stability data is supplied an applicant is asked to give an assurance of on-going stability testing to the end of the product shelf-life.

With regard to Phytopharmaceuticals, a new annex will be added to the fresh revision of the UK guideline. Guidance on phytopharmaceuticals or "herbals" as they are called in the UK, is currently available in a small separate guideline entitled "Mal 39 – Products containing Herbal Ingredients". It is this which is being revised and updated to become a new annex in the main guideline.

9. Conclusion

The requirements of the UK Licensing Authority on stability testing are largely consistent with the requirements of the European Council Directives. The UK Licensing Authority recognises and accepts data from other countries provided that they are consistent with UK requirements. With regard to EC Member States, the CPMP is working towards a common standard guideline through its working party on quality matters. This may take about 2 years to complete.

In concluding a consideration of stability testing it is important to remember what was quoted at a seminar in Geneva in 1976 on the Stability of Pharmaceutical Products, namely, that,

> Stability is not all
> but all comes to naught
> without stability.

References

(1) The Medicines Act 1968 and its various Statutory Instruments HMSO (London)
(2) Guidance Notes on Applications for Product Licences (formerly MAL 2) HMSO (London)
(3) Guidance Notes on Applications for Clinical Trial Certificates and Clinical Trial Exemptions (formerly MAL 2 and MAL 62) HMSO (London)
(4) Int. J. Pharm. Tech. and Prod. Mfr., 3 (2) 43–46, 1982

XI. Stability and Stability Testing of Medicinal Products

APV-Guidelines and Commentary

1. APV Guideline

1.1 Application and Purpose

These guidelines are applicable to drugs manufactured for use on or in humans or animals which are introduced to the market in a packaged form suitable for supply to the consumer (drug products).

They provide

● A definition of the term "Stability."
● A summary of storage conditions.
● A description of the principles of stability testing.

These guidelines can just give the general principles and they must be modified for each drug product depending on the extent and type of the stability testing to be undertaken and the available resources.

1.2 Definition of Stability

Stability means compliance with the quality, as defined in the specifications of a product, up to the end of the shelf life laid down by the manufacturer.

The quality of a drug product is determined by its content of active ingredient, its purity and organoleptic, physicalchemical and microbiological properties.

1.2.1 Content of Active Ingredient

Unless governed by other regulations (e.g. Pharmacopoeias, EEC-Directives), the assay of the active ingredient of a drug product should not fall below 90 % of the label claim up to the end of the shelf life.

This tolerance limit applies to stored products and must be confirmed by results of suitable stability tests. For freshly manufactured products (i.e., finished product at the end of the manufacturing cycle), the permitted deviation limits of $\pm 5\%$ may not be exceeded without appropriate justification (1).

1.2.2 Purity, Degradation Products

Degradation products should be identified and limited wherever possible. Adequate assurance must be available that degradation products do not lead to an increase in toxicity of the drug product concerned.

1.2.3 Organoleptic, Physico-Chemical and Microbiological Properties

The quality of the drug product with respect to the organoleptic, physico-chemical and microbiological properties is considered assured if

- the results of the stability test conform to the specifications,
- the drug product can be used as directed,
- any changes that occur are not so pronounced that consumer acceptance is impaired.

1.3 Stability Overage

The stability overage is that amount of an active ingredient which is added in excess of the declared content to compensate for loss of active ingredient during storage.

Generally, the stability overage should not exceed 10 % of the declared content. In certain cases, exceptions are permitted when the stability is less than three years.

1.4 Storage Time, Shelf-Life

The storage time or shelf-life is that period of time during which the quality of a drug product, if stored correctly, is assured, i.e., compliance with specifications is present.

A use life, and if necessary storage instructions, must be given for drug products which are reconstituted into a usable form directly before administration or whose stability is jeopardized once the container is opened. The use life is that period of time for which a drug product may be used by the consumer once the container has been opened or the product has been reconstituted directly before use.

Shelf-life and use life must be determined experimentally.

1.5 Storage Conditions

Storage is understood to mean maintaining the product for a longer period of time under normal or defined conditions.

1.5.1 Normal Storage Conditions

Storage in dry, well-ventilated rooms at room temperature with the exclusion of extraneous odours, other forms of contamination and intense light. Room temperature according to the European Pharmacopoeia is 15 °C–25 °C, according to the USP, 15 °C–30 °C.

Drug products which can be stored under these conditions require no special storage instructions.

1.5.2 Defined Storage Conditions

Drug products which must be stored under defined conditions require appropriate storage instructions.

Unless otherwise specifically stated, e. g., continous maintenance of cold storage, the respective directions do not need to be observed during short-term interruptions, for example, during transportation.

The following instructions should be used:

"Do not store over 30 °C."	(from + 2 °C to + 30 °C)
"Do not store over 25 °C."	(from + 2 °C to + 25 °C)
"Do not store over 20 °C."	(from + 2 °C to + 20 °C)
"Do not store over 8 °C."	(from + 2 °C to + 8 °C)
"Do not store below 8 °C."	(from + 8 °C to + 25 °C)
"Protect from moisture."	

(no more than 60 % relative humidity at room temperature)
"Protect from light."

1.5.3 Labeling

Storage instructions for healthcare professionals are to be placed in readily visible places and in clearly legible form on the containers of the drug product and on any outer wrappings.

Storage instructions for the user are to be given in the package insert.

1.6 Packaging

Packaging is the total of all packaging materials, consisting of the container, its closure (these two form the primary packaging) as well as any outer wrapping and the package insert with which the drug product is marketed and/or stored.

The packaging should protect the drug product from prejudicial effects such as light, air, moisture and mechanical wear and tear.

1.7 Stability Testing

Stability testing is the basis for, among other things, the selection and establishment of suitable container/closure systems, the shelf-life, the use life, storage and the directions for storage for the respective drug product.

The shelf-life of a drug product is established from the stability tests carried out on the finished product. The formulation of the product tested must be identical with that to be marketed. Batches of a similar composition made during development phase may be included in the evalultion.

1.7.1 Container und Closure

During the stability tests, the drug is to be stored in the same container/closure system as that in which the drug product is to the marketed.

Projections regarding the stability in other containers and closures are only valid if it is shown that these are at least as good, if not better, than those already tested.

1.7.2 Accelerated Studies

In such studies, the samples to be investigated are stored under stress conditions. The results of accelerated stability testing can be used in the prediction of stability.

1.7.3 Long-Term Studies

Stability tests are based on long-term studies, the results of which are used to derive the shelf life for individual countries or climatic zones.

1.7.3.1 Storage Conditions for Long-Term Studies

The storage conditions (temperature, relative humidity) for the samples to be tested must be defined for long-term studies. The conditions should correspond to the climatic conditions of the various countries or climatic zones in which the drug product is to be stored.

1.7.3.2 Duration of Studies

The samples should be stored for at least the duration of the shelf-life as established by the manufacturer for the respective product.

1.7.3.3 Test Intervals

Since it is recognized that time-related changes in quality can occur in long-term studies, an adequate number of repeat tests must be undertaken at suitable test intervals.

1.7.3.4 Test Criteria

The stability tests can, in principle, be limited to those quality characteristics which can change during storage, transport or proper use of the drug product concerned. The actual selection of the respective test parameters must always be specific to the particular product.

Every stability test plan should, however, include an organoleptic examination, a study of the physical and chemical parameters that define quality, a quantitative determination of the active ingredient and if necessary, a specific test for degradation products and quantitative evaluation of preservatives.

1.7.3.5 Test Methods

The analytical methods used to measure the content of active ingredient must be specific, sensitive, give good reproducibility and/or have been validated.

If no sufficiently specific technique for determining the active ingredient is available, then a test for degradation products is required. The latter test may give additional information especially in accelerated stability tests. Objective evaluation techniques are to be preferred to verbal descriptions for the organoleptic examinations.

1.7.4 On-Going Stability

In order to confirm the results on which the stability is based, it is recommended that even after the particular drug product has been introduced on to the market, the stability of samples from other batches should be tested.

2. Commentary on the APV Guidelines

by Wolfgang Grimm

2.1 Stability and Stability Testing of Drug Products

Drug products can undergo various chemical and physical changes. The active ingredient can decompose, interact with excipients or the primary packaging material or the physical properties can alter. These „instabilities" can be potentiated or induced by temperature stresse moisture, light or oxygen.

Steps must, therefore, be taken to ensure the consumer receives a drug product which is fully effective and safe. To this end, extensive stability studies are necessary with the product in question and where applicable, with its starting materials and intermediates.

A major contribution to the safety of drugs was provided by the publication in 1972 of the APV-Guidelines 23 06 72 on the Stability and Storage of Drug Products.

In the intervening period, the appreciation of the problem has markedly increased, our scientific knowledge has greatly improved and official regulations have been drawn up. For these reasons, the APV-Guidelines have been revised and Stability Testing is now included alongside Stability as a now focal point of interest.

The current version of Stability Guidelines reflects the current state of the art. They basically correspond to current practice in the Federal Republic of Germany both in the conduct of stability tests in the pharmaceutical industry and also in the assessment of stability problems by the authorities. At the same time, the Guidelines enable those engaged in the field of drug stability in other countries to compare their own procedures to measure stability with those in this country. They may thus be a valuable aid in the efforts, so vitally needed, to establish internationally recognized criteria for assessing the quality of drug products.

The Guidelines are intended to be applicable to all drugs in whatever dosage form. They can, therefore, just give the general principles from which the extent and type of testing for each individual case can be derived.

2.2 Definition of Stability

The evaluation of stability of a drug product is concerned with the content of active ingredient, the purity and organoleptic, physical/chemical and if appropriate, the microbiological properties. Stability predictions, therefore, must cover these criteria.

Stability means that the results of tests on a product must lie within the specified tolerance limits right up to the end of the shelf-life. Hence, the establishment of product specifications is particularly important.

If changes do occur during storage, it is recommended that the internal specifications for the release of a batch of freshly manufactured goods are made somewhat tighter.

In the future, the officially permitted limit for the content of active ingredient in the final product at the end of the manufacturing (freshly manufactured products) will be $\pm 5\%$; whereas, a wider limit will be permitted for stored goods which must, nevertheless, be verified by appropriate stability studies (2).

2.2.1 Active Ingredient

Statements on the stability of the active ingredient relate primarily to the therapeutically active ingredients which are present as chemically defined substances. The aim, however, must be to gradually include drugs of botanical origin and other natural substances so that in the future, a uniform standard of quality exists for all drug products.

The stated limits for content of active ingredient (95% or 90%) are more of a theoretical nature for biological products. In many cases, the variability associated with the methods used (e.g., the determination of the activity of sera and vaccines using animal models) means that these limits cannot be maintained. Therefore, the inherent error of the method must be borne in mind when evaluating the results.

Ingredients contributing to the efficacy, such as preservatives or antioxidants, should also be included in the stability test but in such cases, other tolerance limits are applicable. Thus the preservative effect must be assured up to the end of the shelf-life, an antioxidant can be used up at the end of the shelf-life.

2.2.2 *Purity, Degradation Products*

If degradation products are formed, they should be identified whenever possible and their toxicity examined. If the results of toxicity tests show that no limits need to be placed on their content, then degradation can be tolerated provided that the 90% limit for content of active ingredient is maintained. If attempts to identify the degradation products are unsuccessful, then a comparative toxicological study of degraded and non-degraded samples can be conducted to confirm the harmlessness of these.

2.2.3 *Organoleptic, Physico-Chemical and Microbiological Characteristics*

Changes that are organoleptically detectable, particularly in the appearance, are frequently not accompanied by any analytically detectable decrease in the content of the active ingredient. It can, therefore, be advisable to point out that slight changes in the external appearance are harmless. Statistical techniques can be included to evaluate physico-chemical changes.

2.3 *Stability Overage*

A stability overage should not be used to avoid printing an open expiry date or to compensate for inadequate formulation of the product.

2.4 *Stability Period, Shelf-Life*

The results of stability testing should be used to derive the shelf-life of a drug product. This shelf-life should not exceed five years. Giving a shelf-life of longer than five years is generally not considered sensible. Up to the end of the stated shelf-life, the manufacturer guarantees the quality of the product. In the Federal Republic of Germany, the following legal regulations must be observed:

Drug products which were registered before 31.12.1977, according to the old Medicines Act, carry an open expiry date when the stability is less than two years. (This requirement is not taken directly from the AMG 61 – the Medicines Act – but from an official report of the Health Commission.)

Drugs which have been registered since 01.01.1978, according to the new AMG, must, according to section 10, paragraph 7, carry an open expiry date when they are not stable for more than three years.

According to the EEC Directive passed on 26.10.1983, in the future an expiry date must generally be given. This Directive must be incorporated into the national laws of member states within 18 months.

Some drug companies have, in the meantime, adopted the practice of giving an open expiry date for all drug products.

If the drug product is stable for less than one year, calculated from the date it is released to the market by the pharmaceutical company, then the expiry date must be given to the exact day.

In other cases, the 30 June of 31 December of a year is to be given with the date chosen always being the one before the actual expiry date.

The expiry date on the container, and if applicable, on the exterior wrapping, should be given in a clearly legible and durable form.

The use of the words "expiry date" is not stipulated but the phrase "use by..." is recommended.

In order to avoid giving the consumer the impression that a drug product has a reduced therapeutic effect towards the end of its shelf-life, it is recommended that it is pointed out in the package insert that the quality is assured up to the end of the shelf life.

With certain dosage forms, it is necessary to give additional information pertaining to quality over and above the shelf life itself.

Thus for syrups and injections that are supplied in a dry form for reconstitution before administration, information as to the use life of the freshly prepared product (often combined with storage instructions) should be given.

The same applies to tightly closed multidose containers with sterile contents as well as those preparations, the stability of which is affected by the entry of air during the use life.

2.5 Storage Conditions

For the storage of drug products, a differentiation is made between normal storage conditions for which no special instructions are needed and defined storage conditions where specific directions must be given.

In this context, a distinction should also be drawn between storage instructions for professionals, e. g., pharmacists and directions for the user.

Thus, suppositories are generally subject to no special storage instructions because it is known in professional circles that they must not be stored over 30 °C. On the other hand, the user should receive instructions as to storage.

From the results of the stability testing, it can be determined whether a defined storage condition is necessary to ensure the stability of a drug product. Relevant instructions must be unambiguous, clear and practicable.

Since the maintenance of storage instructions always entails expenditure, it is important to critically examine whether or not they are needed. For example, the instruction "Do not store over 20 °C" should only be used if stability tests have shown that the stability on storage under normal conditions in termperature ranges of between 20 °C and 25 °C cannot be quaranteed.

Storage instructions should not be used to compensate for inadequate galenical development.

2.6 Packaging

A difference is made between the container/closure system (also called the primary packaging) and the outer wrapping. Both from the packaging.

Container and closure are in direct contact with the drug product.

Primary packaging materials and if plastic containers are used, then occasionally even the label can lead to undesirable and unexpected interactions with the drug product itself. The choice of these containers and closures and the reproducibility of their quality should receive particular attention.

2.7 Stability Testing

It is recommended that stability tests are systematically planned and conducted.

Thus a list of requirements should be initially drawn up in which all the criteria which should be covered during the shelf life are listed.

The nature and scope of the stability tests corresponding to the problems associated with the product are then specified in a study plan.

There is thus a difference as to whether the product under consideration is a new active ingredient in a new dosage form, a new dosage form with a known active ingredient, an analogous formulation or a dosage or variant of a known formula.

In conducting stability tests, a distinction is made between accelerated stability tests, long-term shelf studies and ongoing stability tests, for each type of study has its own special objective.

2.7.1 Accelerated Stability Tests

Accelerated stability tests serve to identify the weak points in a formulation, to select the test criteria anc to check the suitability of the analytical techniques.

The results of these investigations provide estimates of shelf-life and predict stability. Accelerated studies are particularly helpful in comparative stability tests. Stability projections from accelerated storage, using data obtained from the reaction kinetics, are only possible when they have been qualified using a mathemetical/statistical treatment.

This requires highly reproducible measurement techniques for the active ingredient or its degradation products and when the Arrhenius Equation is used, an adequately large number of elevated temperatures.

The interpretation of kinetic extrapolations requires special care when applied to heterogeneous liquid and semi-solid systems.

The relative importance assigned to the various phases of stability testing can vary. Thus, increased effort during the accelerated stability testing phase may result in fewer tests being necessary in the subsequent long-term shelf studies if, for example, reliable projections of stability already exists.

The expense of accelerated stability testing is offset by a considerably increased confidence in the stability predictions and a decisive saving in time.

2.7.2 Long-Term Studies

These form the core of stability tests and the mandatory shelf lives are derived from these results.

If worldwide stability information is needed, the following points are important:

● Number and definition of the climatic zones.
● Storage conditions.
● Duration of test and test intervals.

For the pruposes of worldwide stability tests, one can divide the earth into four climatic zones: (3)

Climatic Zones I   – Temperate climate.
Climatic Zone II   – Subtropical and Mediterranean climates.
Climatic Zone III   – Hot, dry climate.
Climatic Zone IV   – Hot, humid climate.

To classify a city or a country in the correct climatic zone standard values, as given in Table 1, are applicable. (4)

In calculating the average annual temperature, all values $< 19\,°C$ when measured in the open are assigned to be $19\,°C$.

The storage conditions appropriate to the individual climatic zones should take account of seasonal variations in climate and if possible, correspond to the actual climatic conditions. They should be definitively established and monitored. Only in this way is it possible to compare individual batches with each other and to draw generally applicable conclusions from pachaging tests.

In "natural," non-controlled and defined storage conditions, there is for example, a tremendous difference depending on whether one stores a batch in summer or winter, relative to the six-month value.

Table 1
Criteria and standard values for assigning a city to the correct climatic zone.

| Criteria | Standard Values for the Various Climatic Zones | | | |
	I	II	III	IV
Average annual temp. measured in the open.	Up to 15°C	15–22°C	> 22°C	> 22°C
Calculated average annual temp. (< 19°C).	Up to 20.5°C	20.5–24°C	> 24°	> 24°
Average annual partial vapor pressure.	Up to 11 mbar	11–18 mbar	Up to 15 mbar	> 15 mbar

The duration of the test is at least as long as the full shelf-life. The test intervals are established as a framework, the actual number of investigations depends, however, on the particular problem itself.

The following factors are important in carrying out the long term studies:

- Number of batches and how they are selected,
- Test criteria,
- Test methods.

The number of batches cannot be generally specified. This depends on the type of problem and the nature of the information on the product.

The selection of samples must be undertaken with great care, it must be representative of the manufacturing process.

Samples of batches manufactured to the final formulation and in the same container/closure system as that in which the drug product is to be marketed form the basis on which statements concerning stability are made.

Valuable information is, however, also obtained from the results of studies with variations on this formulation or analogous formulations which display the same or similar stability characteristics. This also applies to the container/closure system.

If positive test data for a critical primary packaging material are available, then a less critical one can be assessed by analogy, e. g., blister pack PVC 250 um and PVC/PVDC foil laminates.

Those quality characteristics which can be particularly significant for quality or acceptance and which can change on storage should be selected as test criteria.

Tolerances to identify significant changes compared to the initial value (predictive ability of the method) and limits of tolerance for changes that do occur should be known. Tolerance limits have a decisive influence on the quality and shelf-life of drug products.

2.7.3 Ongoing Studies

By carrying out ongoing studies on batches from the current production, stability predictions checked and statistically confirmed.

References

(1) From the EEC Council of Ministers Amendment of 26.10.83 to the Directives 65/65/EEC, 75/318/EEC and 75/319/EEC on the approximation of provisions laid down by law, regulation or administrative action relating to proprietary drug products. Official Journal of the European Communities No. L 332/5, November 28, 1983.
(2) See Footnote 1, page 2.
(3) Futscher, N., Schumacher, P., Pharm. Ind. 34, 479–483 (1972)
(4) Grimm, W., Pharm. Ind. 47, 981–985, 1082–1089 (1985)

XII. APV-Guidelines: Stability and Stability Testing

State of the art in the field of stability and stability testing
W. Oeser, Hamburg

This contribution is not concerned with requirements of any licensing or watchdog authority, nor with conditions or demands from one particular side, instead it is hoped to show that the Guidelines under discussion are intended to offer some assistance to all involved in this field, but especially to those directly engaged in stability testing. It is not the views of the regulatory bodies which are represented by these Guidelines, but rather those of the pharmaceutical industry.

What we are dealing with is a document that provides a comprehensive description of the problems encountered in stability and stability testing and which is based – and this is extremely important for the proper appreciation of the Guidelines – on the broadest conceivable consensus of expert opinion.

It should be emphasised at the very outset that the Guidelines are about the accepted state of the art in the field of stability and stability testing.

This term "state of the art" or "generally acknowledged current stage of development or knowledge" deserves some further consideration, but first some fundamental points about guidelines need to be explained.

- What force do guidelines of a general nature actually possess?
- Who uses them?
- How are they drawn up and when can one speak of "accepted" guidelines?
- What is their relationship to compulsory statutory regulations?

We live in an age of rules and regulations. The streets have become so congested with vehicles that detailed traffic laws are necessary to regulate traffic flow and ensure road safety.

The obvious requirements of quality, efficacy and lack of toxicity are alone not sufficient to ensure a proper supply of drugs to the public. Instead a law is needed, which, through its provisions, looks after safety in the drugs market. But even these provisions are not enough to settle questions of detail, especially those of a technical nature. The legislator therefore allows the executive branch to resolve such questions (within a previously established framework) by subordinate legislation. In-depth knowledge of the subject is needed on the part of the executive to translate the intention of the legislator into practicable possibilities. We all realize that compromises must be made here. Nevertheless, or perhaps because of this, the more detailed the legislation is in scientific terms, the more strongly the legislator and the executive tend to base their standards and requirements on the current state of scientific knowledge, without themselves knowing this state in all its details.

Numerous examples of this situation exist:

The Regulations Governing the operation of Pharmaceutical Companies state that drugs must be manufactured in accordance with accepted pharmaceutical principles (1). Naturally, the legislator is not in a position – and according to our understanding of the law – is not called upon, to elaborate and specify either general or detailed manufacturing instructions. He restricts himself to emphasizing that the process is to be undertaken according to generally recognized pharmaceutical principles. The subordinate legislation is accompanied by an official interpretation, which is no longer legally binding, but is primarily a commentary by the executive itself and states that the Pharmacopoeia in particular, is to be counted among the sources of accepted pharmaceutical principles. (That is actually not completely consistent or logical, since the Pharmacopoeia itself represents a legally binding standard work and has thus lost the character of a guideline).

More consistent are the Regulations Governing the Operation of Pharmacies. These stipulate that drugs are to be prepared in accordance with the requirements of the Pharmacopoeia and that if the Pharmacopoeia itself does not contain any instructions regarding manufacture, then generally recognised rules of the pharmaceutical sciences are to be applied (2). The regulations name the German Pharmaceutical Codex (DAC), in addition to the (binding) Pharmacopoeia, as a scientific source of guidance. One may therefore assume that the directions of the DAC are regarded by the executive as generally accepted rules of pharmaceutical science.

And a third example: The application for licensing a drug product with the appropriate Federal German Authority must include details of the method used to ensure stability, the duration of stability, the method of storage and the results of the stability tests. The licensing authority is provided with general directives on standards, which must correspond to the prevailing state of scientific knowledge and be constantly updated to conform to this (3).

Further examples can be freely cited. The three given here merely illustrate that in many cases, one refers back to the state of the art.

It would certainly be tempting sometime to determine whether different phrases such as

- accepted pharmaceutical principles
- the generally recognized rules of pharmaceutical science
- the prevailing state of scientific knowledge

really mean different things.

It is assumed here that all formulations have the same aim namely to refer to that which is usually regarded by experts in the field as feasible, necessary and proper.

The real problem is to ensure that where reference is made to the state of the art, then knowledge of this state must be made available to everyone. The executive do not determine what is in accordance with the rules, but simply require that the rules are conformed with, so that it can be stipulated that conformity is to be used as the standard. The state of the art must therefore be describable and even legally evaluable. This is where the APV Guidelines can be useful with regard to questions on stability and stability tests.

The more closely guidelines fulfill the criterion of describing the latest state of technology, or the so-called state of the art, the more the guidelines (although not legally binding) will be accepted and regarded as a valuable and significant report. Lawyers formulate it like this:

"Rules to technology are regarded as generally established if their theoretical principles are known and accepted by a majority of scientists (specialists) and if they are known and recognised as correct by leading circles involved in their practical application" (4).

Knowledge and acceptance are thus the decisive criteria.

It is quite clear from their past history that these newly revised Guidelines fill a definite need. They are based on the APV Guidelines of 1972 (5), which have been cited in almost all publications on stability since that time. Thus the work of the APV in this field is well known and perhaps one may say is widely accepted as coming from a renowned organisation.

According to the constitution of the APV, the task of this association is to support pharmaceutical technology and quality control in drug manufacture in scientific and practical ways, with the aim of optimising the dosage form and increasing drug safety. Among the ways of achieving this aim is indeed the drawing up of guidelines and working aids. (Quote from the constitution of the association).

It may therefore be assumed that the profession at large attaches great importance to the guidelines of the APV – although they are so far few in number.

Nevertheless, the APV has not made light of the task of preparing these revised Guidelines. The APV has worked on them internally for many years, has discussed and revised the draft and then circulated a further draft within the professional public. These experts accepted the invitation to comment, their views were heeded and the draft was once again extensively and systematically revised before the paper, with the Commentary by Dr. Grimm, was finally adopted in the autumn of 1984 (6).

The Guidelines are directed principally to specialists in the field of stability, but also to interested members of the general public. They begin by providing definitions, then deal in the second part, with storage conditions and in the third, describe the principles of stability testing.

The terms defined are:

- Stability
- Content of active ingredient
- Purity, degradation products
- Organoleptic, physicochemical and
  microbiological characteristics
- Stability overages
- Period of stability, shelf-life and stability after opening.

The central definition in all this, is that of stability. All other expressions merely serve to explain this central term further.

Stability is defined as the maintenance of the quality defined in the specification of the drug until the end of the manufacturer's stated shelf-life. The new definition no longer refers to an absolute quality as in the 1972 Guidelines. At that time, one was geared towards constant content of active ingredient and unchanged galenical condition (absolute terms!). Today the definition is relative (quality as defined in the specification until the end of the manufacturer's stated shelf-life) and this takes more account of the actual relationships of a constantly changing system.

On the other hand, the specification parameters have become wider, have been differentiated and now include

- Content of active ingredient
- Purity
- Organoleptic characteristics
- Physicochemical
- Microbiological criteria.

By this means, interested members of the public also gain an impression of the complexity of the problems.

At the same time, the public also receives concrete assistance in its contacts with drugs, as now a clear distinction is drawn between periods of stability on the one hand for the drug product in unchanged form, and stability after opening (which is directed at those handling and using drug products). In the interests of drug safety, it is to be hoped that in future, greater use will be made than hitherto of this way of providing proper information for the consumer. The same applies to the differentiation of storage instructions primarily for health care professionals and principally relating to the unopened product, and those instructions directed at the consumer, which generally relate to opened packs. In the latter case, account has to be taken of entirely predictable problems or risks posed by well-known mishandling of drugs by the consumer, which can be overcome through practically-orientated information.

The third focus of attention of the paper arises from the change in the title of the Guidelines.

Whereas the 1972 Guidelines were headed:

"Stability and Storage of Drugs"

the title now reads

"Stability and Stability Testing of Drugs".

It is rightly assumed that stability tests form the basis for the selection and establishment of

- suitable containers and closures
- the period of stability
- stability after opening
- storage instructions for professionals and finally
- storage instructions for the consumer.

The Guidelines deal with containers in which the drug should be kept during the storage experiments (stability testing). They mention accelerated stability tests and long term tests and stress that stability testing must extend over the entire shelf life of the respective drug product stated by the manufacturer.

They discuss the key words

- Testing intervals
- Testing criteria
- Testing method and finally
- Follow-up stability.

Nonetheless, these Guidelines can only give advice, discuss the matter, draw attention to criteria and show broad principles. They cannot replace the construction of a Test Protocol, which has to be individually drawn up for each drug preparation.

Dr. Grimm, in his already mentioned Commentary, describes the functions of Guidelines as follows:

"The current version of the stability guidelines reflects the present state of knowledge. They basically correspond to current practice in the Federal Republic of Germany, both in the execution of stability tests in the pharmaceutical industry and also in the assessment of questions of stability by the authorities. At the same time, the Guidelines enable those engaged in stability problems in other lands to compare their own measures to ensure stability with those in our country. They can thus be a valuable aid in the vitally necessary efforts to establish internationally recognised criteria for the evaluation of drug quality" (7). Nothing further need be added.

References

(1) Gesetzblatt der Bundesrepublik Deutschland (Bundes-Gesetzblatt I of 15. March 1985, page 546)
(2) 7 of the Verordnung über Betrieb von Apotheken of 7. August 1968 (Bundesgesetzblatt I page 939)
(3) Gesetz über den Verkehr mit Arzneimitteln vom 24. August 1976 (Bundesgesetzblatt I, page 2445, 26)
(4) von Heymann, E.: Arzneimittelprüfung nach dem jeweiligen Stand der wissenschaftlichen Erkenntnisse. Pharm. Ztg. 1974, 1901
(5) APV Guidelines 230 0672
(6) Pharm. Ind. 47, 6, 627 (1985)
(7) Ibid.

XIII. Stability Testing in Industry

Wolfgang Grimm, Analytik, Dr. Karl Thomae GmbH, D-Biberach

1. Introduction

The drugs of today, which are almost exclusively manufactured in industry, must be able to withstand transport and storage over long periods.

In these respects they differ markedly from those of earlier times, which were prepared in pharmacies for immediate use and whose perfect quality merely had to be ensured up to the end of treatment.

However the full effectiveness of drugs industrially manufactured in large batches must be guaranteed right up to the end of the declared shelf-life. This can only be ensured by extensive investigations, the Stability Tests.

These Stability Tests have nowadays become an integral part of the steps Industry takes to safeguard the quality of drug products.

As progress in pharmaceutical technology and therapeutics has enabeled advances to be made in the manufacture and use of drugs, so Stability Testing, has in the course of time, developed into an interdisciplinary science. It can thus only fulfill its task if, in addition to analytical criteria, pharmaceutical-technological, biochemical and in future, also biotechnological criteria are taken into account.

In Industry, Stability Testing pursues two particular aims;

– Determination of the optimum formulation during pharmaceutical-technological development
– Derivation of the stability of a product, which guarantees the full activity of the drug up to the end of its shelf-life.

The declared stability derived from the results of the Stability Tests represents a comprehensive assessment of quality, including organoleptic, physico-chemical, chemical and, if appropriate, microbiological criteria. It applies to all batches.

The results of Stability Testing

– provide the means by which the patient can be guaranteed perfect quality
– from the basis of Registration and Licensing Documents
– provide information for professionals such as hospital and retail pharmacists.

The importance of Stability Testing will increase still further with the forthcoming general open expiry dating in the EEC. It is the declared aim of Industry

– to develop products with the longest possible stability, the target is 5 years,

– to optimise pharmaceutical-technological development to such a degree that storage instructions can be dispensed with wherever possible,
– not to use minimum stability dates, but to give shelf lives, based on scientific tests.

2. Conduct of Stability Tests

Stability Testing in Industry covers a wide area due to:

– Different product programmes
– Different marketing objectives, sales in one country, one climatic zone or worldwide.

This results in a multitude of various Stability Programmes which nonetheless share a series of common principles, which will now be described. At the same time it will be shown,

– what outlay is necessary in industry's view,
– what degree of certainty lies behind the declarations of stability.

Among the route from new drug substance to full scale production, 6 phases in Stability Testing can be distinguished: (1)

– Tests with the drug substance
– Screening during pharmaceutical development
– Accelerated Studies with chosen formulations
– Long Term Testing
– Follow-up Studies
– Tests after alterations to routine production

The full Stability Test Programme will be performed only, when it begins with a new drug substance.
If the development however starts with a new dosage form of a known drug substance Stability Testing begins with phase two. Does it start with a new dose level or a parallel development Stability Testing begins with Accelerated Studies or Long Term Studies.
The various tests within these 6 phases must be closely coordinated,

– so that the state of information about a product is being constantly updated,
– so that reliable declarations of stability can be derived as soon as possible.
– to ensure that the outlay is in reasonable proportion to the result obtained

Now in order to determine the outlay and effort required for each of the phases in drug development and for stability tests in general, the following procedure is adopted:

– The particular problem is specified by narrowly defining the objective.

– A profile of the required characteristics is drawn up in which all the factors to be addressed by the stability declaration are listed.
– A check is made as to how far these factors are already covered by existing results.
– A Testing Plan is produced which establishes the required outlay and design.

The Testing Plan contains the following instructions:

– Storage conditions
– Testing criteria
– Testing methods
– Samples
– Number of batches
– Duration of Test
– Testing Intervals

Finally, the results which must cover the profile of required characteristics are summarised.

This approach clearly indicates that the effect and extent ought to be matched to the particular problem under consideration.

3. Description of the individual phases in a Stability Testing Programme

Starting with a new drug substance

3.1 Tests with the drug substance

Purpose

Determination of the Stability Profile of the drug substance

Required Characteristics

Listing of the factors which can affect the stability of the drug substance during handling or storage such as: Temperature, humidity, air, light, pH.
  Statements concerning solubility and polymorphism are given here.
  These tests are not orientated towards any dosage forms.

Testing Plan

Storage conditions:	Corresponding to the influencing factors to be considered, e.g. high temperature
Testing criteria:	Appearance, content, degradation

Testing methods: Stability-specific
Samples: Representative of batches of drug substance
Duration of Test: Up to 3 months
Testing Intervals: Variable, depending on the stability behaviour
Evaluation of results: Construction of the Stability Profile containing details of the stability behaviour and, if appropriate, instructions for handling, storage and possible dosage forms corresponding to test results

3.2 Screening during pharmaceutical development

This phase includes pharmaceutical or galenical development from the first preliminary studies up to the final formulation.

Purpose

– Selection of the optimal formulation
– Determination of the factors affecting stability.

Required characteristics

Listing of the possible internal and external influencing factors e.g. excipients, packaging materials, temperature, humidity, air, light and other criteria relevant to the dosage form. Naturally, any existing results are evaluated before the Testing Plan is drawn up.

Testing Plan

Storage conditions: Corresponding to external factors such as high temperature, humidity, light
Testing criteria: Appearance, relevant physico-chemical parameters, content of drug, degradation
Testing methods: Stability-specific, qualitative only, as far as possible
Samples: Made up of representative drug and excipient batches
Duration of Test: Up to 3 months
Testing Intervals: Variable, depending on the stability behaviour
Evaluation of results: Determination of optimal formulation through data comparison, identification of stability-limiting factors.

Clinical trials also take place during this phase of development and the product samples provided for the trials must also be subjected to stability tests so that their quality during use can be guaranteed. Useful indications of the quality are naturally obtained from the stability profile of the drug substance and the results of screening.

3.3 Accelerated Studies with the chosen formulation

The aim of this phase is to determine whether the formulation selected from Sreening is not only stable in comparison with other variants, but also stable enough in absolute terms for introduction into the market.

Purpose

– Confirmation of the Testing Methods
– Identification of the weak points in the formulation
– Identification of stability-limiting parameters
– Identification of potential problems which could arise during storage and above all, during transport
– Derivation of tentative shelf lives
– Selection of suitable packaging materials

Required characteristics

Listing of potential factors which could influence stability during storage and transport. These include, for example, extremes of temperature, variations in temperature, humidity, light, air.

The Accelerated Studies must be very carefully thought out and planned since absolute statements concerning stability depend on their results. The establishment of relevant storage conditions and the choice of packaging material are especially critical.

Testing for chemical stability is thus carried out in the temperature range of 40–80°C (2).

With solid dosage forms it must be remembered that desorption occurs at high temperatures, even at high relative humidity (3).

If one wishes to evaluate Accelerated Studies in terms of reaction kinetics, then only packaging materials imperious to moisture should be used with solid dosage forms.

For testing for organoleptic and physico-chemical changes storage conditions are selected specifically for the particular dosage form.

For example, for solid dosage forms, the open storage at the conditions of the long Term Testing is suitable.

For semisolid forms −10°C and cycling temperature between 4°C and 40°C.
For liquid forms −10°C.

Testing Plan

Storage conditions	Elevated Temperatures (40–80 °C)
	Temperature cycling (4 °C–40 °C)
	Extreme temperature (−10 °C)
	Those of the Long Term Testing
Testing criteria:	Organoleptic and physico-chemical, relevant to the dosage form
	Content of drug
	Content of any preservatives
	Degradation
	In particular, the frequent quantitative determination of significant degradation products
Testing methods:	Stability specific
Duration of Test:	Up to 3 months
Testing Intervals:	Variable, depending on stability, but at least 4 determinations of content, including initial analysis.

Evaluation of Results:

– Check for significant changes
– Identification of stability-limiting parameter, with proposed tolerance where appropriate
– Derivation of provisional shelf lives using statistics and reaction kinetics (1, 4, 5, 6, 7)
– Establishment of Testing criteria for the Long Term Testing
– Structural identification of significant degradation products (3–10 % at room temperature according to prediction)
– Details of suitable packaging materials

The development phases 2.2 and 2.3 are, in practice, often not so sharply separated as described here.

3.4 Long Term Testing

This phase covers the transition from the laboratory to production scale. It forms the actual core of stability testing, especially as rigorous Accelerated Studies cannot be undertaken with all dosage forms.

Purpose

– Confirmation of the results of the preliminary and Accelerated Studies
– Derivation of binding shelf-lives for the countries and climatic zones where it is planned to market the product
– Derivation of storage instructions, where necessary

Required characteristics

The influencing factors to be examined can be subdivided as follows (8):

Factors from manufacture up to the time of use. Statements concerning the effects of duration of storage, sensitivity to temperature, humidity, light and air, belong here.

These factors can influence stability during:

– Manufacture
– Storage at the manufacturer
– Transport
– Storage at the wholesaler
– Storage in the retail or hospital pharmacy
– Storage in the patient's medicine cupboard at home

Factors influencing stability during use:

– Repeated opening of multidose containers
– Repeated withdrawal from multidose containers.

In a systematically executed Stability Test Programme, a large proportion of these factors can be covered by results already obtained from other investigations.

Testing Plan

In view of the central importance of the Long Term Testing, the individual points of the Testing Plan will be dealt with in detail.

Storage conditions:

Storage conditions must be chosen very carefully; one must be quite clear as to which conditions one wishes to simulate. This applies especially to manufacturers of drugs for export. One cannot include the respective room temperatures for every single country, but must devise a scheme and standardise. In a Stability Test Programme geared to worldwide marketing of a product, the earth is divided into four climatic zones (9) and a realistic storage condition determined for each zone.

These storage conditions should cover the climatic influencing factors to which the drug is exposed in the various climatic zones. That means seasonal and daily

Climatic Zone	Calculated			Derived Storage Condition		
	T (°C)	R.H. (%)	P (mbar)	T (°C)	.R.H. (%)	P (mbar)
I	19.7	43.9	10.0	21	45	11.2
II	22.3	52.9	14.2	25	60	19
III	26.9	31.5	11.1	31	40	18
IV	27.0	78	27.9	31	70	31.5

variations. In addition, they should take into account the official definitions of room temperature, such as:

Ph. Eur. 15–25 °C

USP   15–30 °C

As was shown in one study (10), the following storage conditions can be used, which have been derived from measured climatic values:

Even with a Stability Test Programme geared to worldwide use, storage at 31 °C/40 % R. H. can be omitted. However it is recommended that storage in a refrigerator is also tested and at one stress temperature 41 °C.

– Testing criteria:

Those criteria of a product are examined which,
- during the course of storage may undergo a change
- have a particular significance for quality, effectiveness or acceptance.

– Testing methods and techniques:

The testing methods must ensure that all changes that occur in any of the criteria are unequivocally recorded. The methods used to measure content must be specific and validated. That means the following points should be observed:
- Specificity
- Linearity
- Sensitivity
- Accuracy, recovery rate
- Precision
- Limit of detection

The physical and physioco-chemical techniques should be as detailed as possible.

For the evaluation of organoleptic changes, objective rather then verbal descriptions should be employed wherever this is feasible.

In the assessment of physico-chemical criteria, statistics can be used to help in the evaluation, since repeated measurements are generally taken.

– Selection of batches, stored samples:

Laboratory, pilot-plant and production batches must be representative of manufacture and packaging and should, if possible, come from a validated manufacturing process.

The sample stored must be representative of the batch. The respective samples for analysis must be removed and treated in such a way that the result is representative for the batch at the time of analysis.

– Number of batches:

If it is a new drug substance in a new dosage form, as is described here, then 2–3 batches are required, of different sizes if possible.

If however it is a parallel development or a formulation variant, then 1 to 2 batches suffice.

- Duration of Test:
  Over the entire shelf-life, that is up to a maxiumum of 5 years.
- Testing Intervals:
  The basis for Testing Intervals is given by a set pattern, with testing after 0, 3, 6, 12, 24, 36, 48, 60 months. This can however be adapted if necessary to suit the actual problem under consideration.
- Evaluation of Results:
  Firstly each batch is checked to see whether the results show that any statistically significant changes have occurred in comparison with the initial values at the start of storage. Then the results of the various batches are compared with each other to determine whether, for example, the size of the batch affects stability.

  If a uniform picture emerges, then comprehensive stability data can be derived from the results.

Once again the results are analysed with the help of statistics and reaction kinetics. This is particularly important if the product has not yet been stored for as long as the proposed shelf-life.

The declaration of stability includes all the testing criteria. The shelf-life-limiting parameter is the first one to reach, or which will reach, the tolerance limit specified in the Test Protocol.

If samples are stored under several different conditions corresponding to a Stability Test Programme geared to worldwide marketing, then in the case of stable products, binding stability predictions can be derived after only 6 months (11).

In all cases, this is possible after 12 months.

This applies particularly if the results show good agreement with the preliminary tests and Accerlerated Studies. It means that the test results must lie within the tolerance limits laid down in the Test Protocol up till the end of the shelf-life indicated from these studies, that the quality is guaranteed.

The results from other dosage forms of the same drug substance or those of an analogous formulation may also be drawn upon in deriving or supporting a declaration of stability. The outlay can, in many cases, thereby be significantly reduced. These results are brought together in a Stability Report.

This contains the shelf lives for the various climatic zones, if necessary, a list of suitable packaging materials and where required, instructions concerning storage.

In addition, the report shows all the data that were used to derive stability. Finally, the results are commented upon in terms of organoleptic, physico-chemical, chemical and microbiological properties. The Report must clearly show how the values for stability were derived and verified, by what criteria they are limited and whether they might be extended in the light of future results.

3.5. Follow-up Studies

After at least one representative production batch is stored and tested in the Long Term Testing, further production is subjected to Follow-up Studies.

Purpose

Monitoring of routine production, to see if the shelf lives derived in the Development Phase have continuing validity.

One of the things investigated in the Long Term Study is whether the size of the batch affects stability. If this is not the case, then no markedly deviating results should occur during routine production either. This applies particularly with room temperature storage where storage times = shelf-life.

For this reason, two methods can be used to carry out the Follow-up Studies:

– Investigation of samples stored at room temperature or defined climatic conditions after the end of the shelf-life.
– Investigation of samples which are stored for 6 months at a high temperature (e. g. stress temperature of the Long Term Testing, e. g. 41 °C or 31 °C).

Testing Plan

– Storage conditions:
   ● Room temperature with recording of temperature and relative humidity or defined storage condition
   ● Stress temperature corresponding to Long Term Testing
– Testing criteria:
   Same as Long Term Testing with emphasis on shelf-life-limiting parameter
– Testing methods:
   Stability-specific as in Long Term Testing
– Selection of batches:
   Representative production batch
– Number of batches:
   Dependent on stability of the product. At least one batch per year per storage condition
– Duration of Test:
   Room Temperature: Corresponding to shelf-life
   Stress Temperature: 6 months
– Testing Intervals:
   Initial value, value at end of study
– Evaluation of Results:
   Comparison of results with those of the Long Term Testing

If significantly different results are obtained, then more intensive investigations should be undertaken. If necessary, shortening of the shelf-life.

3.6 Tests after alterations to routine production

If it is necessary to change the manufacturing technique, the composition or the colourants, or to use different packaging materials, then consideration must be given as to whether this is likely to affect stability. The results of the Development Phase can be used as a help in making this decision.

If further stability tests are required, then short term accelerated tests are undertaken in which old and new formulations are compared.

Purpose

Demonstration of whether a different formulation displays a change in stability behaviour.

Testing Plan

- Storage conditions: Elevated temperature as in Accelerated Studies
- Testing criteria: Corresponding to Long Term Testing
- Testing methods: Stability-specific
- Samples: One batch each of the old and new formulation
- Duration of Test: Up to 6 months
- Testing Interval: Corresponding to stability behaviour, however
                                   at least 4 tests including initial value
- Evaluation of Results:
    Comparison of data from the old and new form. If they show no significant differences in stability, then the previous declaration of stability also applies to the new form. Its stability is then monitored in the Follow-up Studies. If the new form is clearly less stable, then the shelf-lives must be correspondingly shortened.

4. Critical Assessment of Stability Test Programmes

If one now subjects the procedures described above to a critical assessment, then one can say that a systematically conducted Stability Test Programme based on scientific knowledge and using methods which correspond to the current state of technology, provides highly reliable declarations of stability.

This is all the more likely to be achieved if the outlay and scope in each phase of the Programme is made appropriate to the particular problem under study.

Naturally, in practice drug development does not always run so smoothly and logically as was shown in the 6 phases. Overlaps or parallel procedures can arise, but the various elements will always be included. The overall Stability Test Programme described here applies to a new dosage form with a new drug substance.

If however, it is

- a new dosage form of a known drug substance
- a new dose level
- a parallel development

then naturally the work involved can be greatly reduced if the results of a systematically conducted stability test are already available. This is reflected in the actual Testing Plan.

5. Cooperation with the Authorities

Stability Tests are undertaken by a manufacturer as a consequence of his responsibility for the satisfactory quality of his drug. The results also form the basis for registration and licensing applications and are therefore examined for their relevance by the appropriate Authorities.

In an attempt to create a uniform standard of quality of drugs and to assist the manufacturers in carrying out Stability Tests, some Authorities draw up Guidelines.

Up to now these differ in their concept, requirements and emphasis.

Were all the individual Guidelines to be taken into account in a worldwide-orientated Stability Test Programme, then an enormous effort would be required, with a multitude of parallel tests.

That cannot be the correct way to proceed! The aim must surely be to orientate

Stability Tests along universally accepted principles which,

– take into account scientific discoveries,
– match the effort and scope to the particular problem.

This requires that:

– Guidelines do not represent absolute requirements, but one of several alternatives accepted by the authorities,
– Data elaborated in another country are generally accepted and recognised.

This is based on the premise that Guidelines are founded on a number of common principles, the observance of which enables Stability Data to be accepted by as many countries as possible.

A good attempt at resolving this problem is offered by the Guidelines "Stability and Stability Testing" issued by the APV (International Association for Pharmaceutical Technology) (12).

Having described, in principle, the procedure in Industry, the most important elements ought to be summarised once again.

– Stability Testing must be undertaken throughout the entire lifespan of the product.
– The effort and scope of the tests are matched to the particular problem.
– All pre-existing stability results are included, as far as possible, in the determination of stability.
– The Stability Testing Programme is systematically conducted in a number of phases which have differing points of emphasis. The following aspects are important:

- Storage conditions
- Testing criteria
- Testing methods
- Number of batches
- Samples
- Duration of Test
- Testing Intervals.

- Statistics and the laws of reaction kinetics are useful aids in evaluating the results.
- The statements about stability are founded on a scientifically based conduct of the Stability Test Programme and evaluation of the results.
- Necessary storage instructions should be standardised.

This raises a whole series of points which could serve as the basis for a discussion.

6. The Future of Stability Testing

The quality of todays drugs has reached a high level due to

- the strict use of GMP Guidelines including validation,
- the great advances in analytical techniques
- the systematic execution of Stability Tests.

What still remains to be done?

Physico-chemical changes are at present largely described in phenomenological terms. Real insight into the causes of changes and their consequences is so far lacking.

One important prerequisite is that the necessary technological properties of excipients are identified and their reproducible quality is ensured.

New discoveries in medicine, progress in pharmaceutical technology and bio-chemistry are leading to dosage forms, to pharmaceutical systems – with a greatly improved efficacy. To ensure the quality – the stability of these products, a close collaborative effort with biochemistry is needed and consideration must be paid to pharmacokinetic criteria.

Step by step this will lead to a much better recognition of those criteria which are important for the action of a drug and to which Stability Testing can be orientated.

This purposeful intensification of the work and outlay will be contrasted by a reduction in the samples which have to be analysed. Thus samples will no longer be tested according to a set timetable, but it will be possible to predict when a significant change is likely.

Intensive efforts must also be directed at ensuring that criteria relevant to the stability of phytopharmaceuticals and drugs with natural constituents can be tested.

The classical dosage forms will still occur in the future. However alongside them, the importance of biotechnology and microelectronics will become ever greater, with correspondingly more complicated pharmaceutical systems. Instead of today's attempts to achieve a constant rate of release of drug, release will be individually adaptable thanks to highly miniaturised and completely biodegradable drug systems with preprogrammed and computer-controlled closed control circuits (13). It will be possible to manufacture hormones, enzymes and antibodies using genetic technology.

In order to cope with these advances, the current existing barriers between the different disciplines will have to be broken down, since development, quality control and stability testing will only be feasible if tackled by a joint team, chosen and organised to solve the particular problem.

It is to be hoped the present resources can be used in their entirety to overcome the problems to be faced and that they will not be bound up by formalistic investigations.

To this end, a mutually trusting cooperation with the Authorities is needed, based on a Stability Test carried out according to principles that are accepted by both sides.

References

(1) PMA's joint-PDS Stability Committee, "Stability Concepts", Pharmaceutical Technology, June 1984
(2) Grimm, W.; Schepky, G.; Stabilitatsprüfung in der Industrie, Editio Cantor Verlag, Aulendorf (1980)
(3) Katdare, A. V.; Bavitz, J. F.; Drug Develop. Ind. Pharm. *10*, 1041–1048 (1984)
(4) Grimm, W.; Hugger, J. P.; Neugebauer, I.; Pharm. Ind. *35*, 733–737 (1973)
(5) Grimm, W; Hugger, J. P.; Pharm. Ind. *36*, 437–443 (1974)
(6) Grimm, W.; Pharm. Ind. *40*, 1165–1173 (1978)
(7) Grimm, W.; Pharm. Ind. *41*, 269–274 (1979)
(8) Grimm, W. in Oelschläger H.; Fortschritte in der Arzneimittelforschung, Wissenschaftliche Verlagsgesellschaft mbH, Stuttgart (1984)
(9) Futscher, M.; Schumacher, P.; Pharm. Ind. *34*, 479 (1972)
(10) Grimm, W.; Pharm. Ind. *47*, 981–985, 1082–1089 (1985)
(11) Grimm, W.; Dtsch. Apoth. Ztg. 271–278 (1984)
(12) APV-Richtlinie und Kommentar, Pharm. Ind. *47*, 627–632 (1985)
(13) Speiser, P.; APV Symposium "Auf der Suche nach den Arzneimitteln der Zukunft", Frankfurt, Oct. 1985

XIV. Analytical Methods of Stability Testing for chemically defined Substances

S. Ebel, University of Würzburg

1. Introduction

It is nearly impossible to review instrumental analytical procedures that may be used in stability testing of chemical defined compounds. Most analysts are using high pressure liquid chromatography with uv detection and believe that this is the only way. Therefore I believe it will be of interest to look to HPLC in this paper especially with respect to modern more sophistical detectors but it will be of more interest to look for other methods too. If for instance uv spectrometry will work in this field, this method is less time consuming and has from this point of view advantages in routine analysis if high numbers of analysis are necessary. At the first glance titration procedures seem to be not sufficient for stability testing but in some cases microtitrations may be done with very high prescision. From other electroanalytical techniques polarography or voltammetry at solid state electrodes are rapid methods avoiding separation techniques that may introduce another source of errors. In order to review possibilities and limitations as well as advantages and disadvantages of different analytical procedures as an example the determination of 4-aminophenol as degradation product of acetaminophen (paracetamol) is used throughout this paper. Most of the analytical research has been elaborated for this purpose and will be published in more details otherwise.

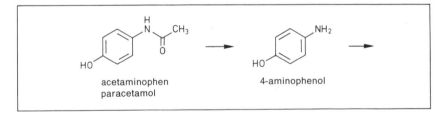

acetaminophen
paracetamol

4-aminophenol

2. High Pressure Liquid Chromatography

The use of high pressure liquid chromatography (HPLC) is state of art in quantitative analysis during stability testing of chemical defined compounds. More than 95

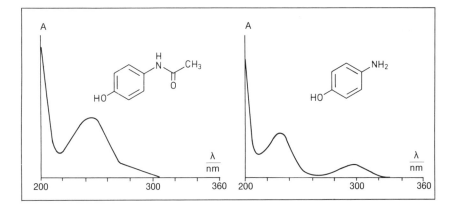

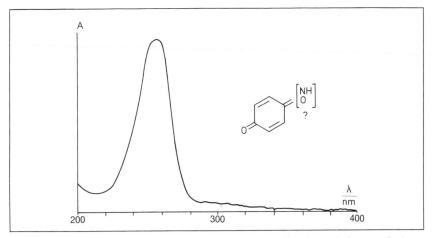

Fig. 1: PAD spectra from HPLC of acetaminophen and its degradation products p-aminophenol and a p-quinone type compound

percent of all analysis in this field are done using normal uv detectors. Therefore the progress caused by modern sophisticated detectors should be of most interest.

Photodiode array detectors (PAD) have the advantage that the uv spectrum of the substance is recorded in less than 50 ms. Using special algorithms for spectral identity it is possible to validate the homogeneity of a HPLC peak. At the other side it is possible by PAD to have an active peak identification and to compare spectra from the running chromatographic process with spectra in a special library (1), (2).

Electrochemical detection (ECD) in HPLC is possible if the separated compounds are oxidized at a glassy carbon electrode as stationary electrode vs a suitable reference electrode (Ag/AgCl): There are two advantages i) higher sensitivity and lower limit of detection; ii) higher selectivity. Both are demonstrated in the choosen example of stability testing of acetaminophen (paracetamol).

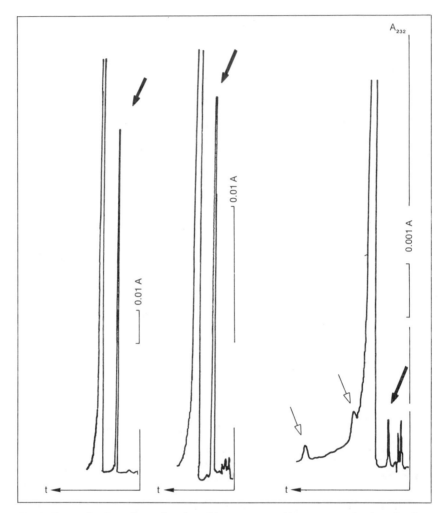

Fig. 2: Determination of p-aminophenol in presence of large amounts of acetaminophen at 232 nm
acetaminophen: 900 ppm
p-aminophenol: 10 ppm
                  1 ppm
                0.1 ppm

Using HPLC with PAD the recorded spectra (fig. 1) are used for identification of
acetaminophen and p-aminophenol. Using p-aminophenol as standard a small
impurity was eluted at higher retention time (fig. 3). This compound was found in
acetaminophen formulations too. Longer storage leads to a definitely higher amount

of this compound. From library uv-spectra in HPLC it is seen that there is a similarity in the spectrum compared to p-quinone, a possible furtheron degradation product.

There is no problem for analysis of acetaminophen by HPLC and uv-detection and a lot of references are found in the literature (cf. (3), (4)). The maximum of absorptivity is at about 245 nm.

Using the maximum of absorptivity of p-aminophenol at 232 nm there is no problem in the analytical HPLC procedure of stability testing of acetaminophen in liquid formulations (fig. 2). In order to have lower limits of detection special procedures of data evaluation may be done to use the whole spectral informations of HPLC with PAD. This shall be demonstrated in the determination of the oxidized 4-aminophenol. The uv spectrum of this compound shows a peak near 254 nm that is very similar to a parabola. From this point of view a convolution operation with a second order orthogonal polynomial centred at 254 nm and using 15 points ($\Delta\lambda$: 240 to 268 nm, $\Delta\lambda = 2$ nm) will enhance the selectivity and increase the sensitivity of determination of this compound. Instead of evaluation of only one absorptivity at the maximum of absorbance the convolution operation uses an integral absorptivity as given by eq. 1 (5).

$$A_{con} = \Sigma A_i \cdot P_i \tag{1}$$

A_i measured absorbance at λ_i
P_i numerical value of orthogonal polynomial

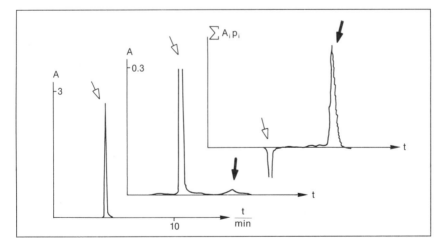

Fig. 3: HPLC of 4-aminophenol and its oxidation product
A: detection at 232 $\pm$ 2 nm
B: same as A but tenfold expansion in absorbance
C: using convolution operation $\lambda_o = 254$ nm, $\Delta\lambda$: 240...268 nm, $\Delta\lambda = 2$ nm

HPLC with electrochemical detection of isomers of aminophenol (6) and of acetaminophen and its metabolites (7) are described in the literature. While p-aminophenol is detected at voltages less than 600 mV vs Ag/AgCl. The ortho-isomer needs about 750 mV and the meta-isomer about 1000 mV. Acetaminophen metabolites are analyzed at 600 mV. In order to find out optimal conditions first the cyclic voltammogrammes had been recorded (fig. 4). Using a glassy carbon working electrode from cyclic voltammogrammes about 160 mV should be applied in analysis of p-amino-phenol resp. 580 mV with acetaminophen.

Optimization with the used electrochemical detector in HPLC leads to about 200 mV in case of p-aminophenol and about 530 mV with acetaminophen to reach the plateau.

From these results it is possible to have a simultaneous determination at 530 mV or a selective detection of the degradation product at 200 mV. The limit of detection

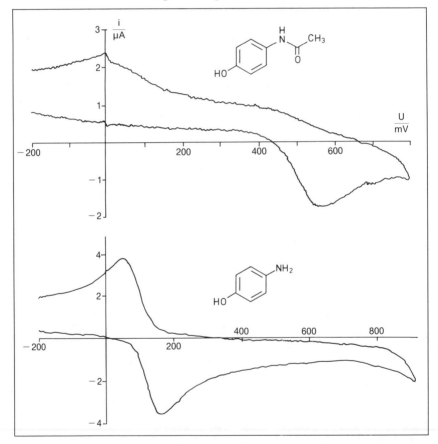

Fig. 4: Cyclic voltammograms of acetaminophen and p-aminophenol als pilote-technique for HPLC with electrochemical detection

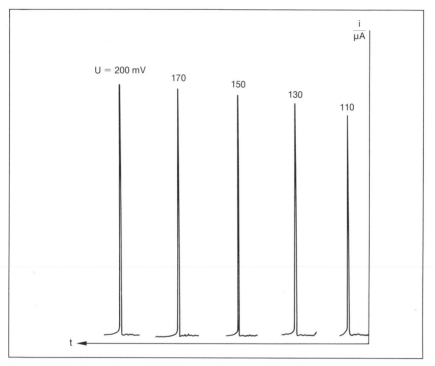

Fig. 5: HPLC optimization of ECD for p-aminophenol (9)

estimated for p-aminophenol is about 5 ppb with a signal to noise ratio of about 7 : 1 (150 mV vs Ag/AgCl) more than sufficient for stability testing of acetaminophen. If the contents of p-aminophenol in acetaminophen is in the order of 1% simultaneous detection at 500 mV is possible (fig. 6), at lower contents the signal of acetaminophen is out of range and the determination has to be done at lower applied voltages (fig. 7) (8).

3. Thin Layer Chromatography

Thin layer chromatography (TLC) is a widespread routine method in qualitative stability testing and it is a very fast method to find out fingerprints of degradation products. Modern computerized instrumental TLC has some advantage in this analytical field. For use in identification uv spectra can be recorded directly from the separated TLC spots. Spectra of the substance absorbed at silicagel are in most cases similar to those obtained in polar solvents, but they are not identically the same. Acetaminophen shows different types of shoulders in the adsorbed state (fig. 8) or in

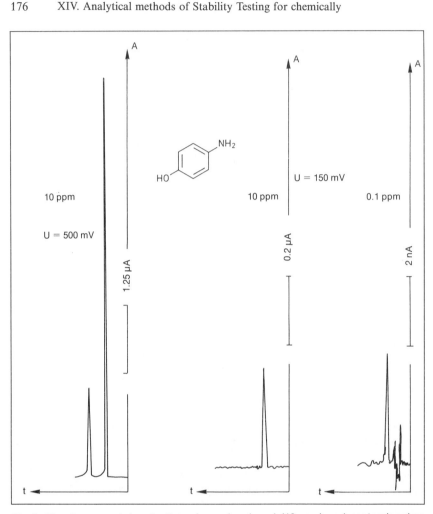

Fig. 6: Simultaneous determination of p-aminophenol (10 ppm) and acetaminophen (900 ppm) at 500 mV applied voltage glassy carbon vs. Ag/AgCl 9

Fig. 7: Determination of p-aminophenol at low amounts at 150 mV applied voltage glassy carbon vs. Ag/Agcl

solution (fig. 1). There are more differences in the spectra of basic or acid drugs as 4-aminophenol.

Using TLC for quantitative analysis in stability testing the solvent has to be elaborated to have maximum separation to detect small amounts of degradation products besides the main substance. For there is no quantitation of the original compound this may eluted near the solvent front. The limit of detection is in TLC not as good as in HPLC for the dynamic range of this method is smaller. To avoid this

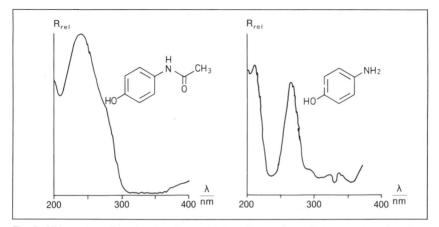

Fig. 8: UV spectra of acetaminophen and its primary degradation product 4-amino-phenol separated by TLC Camag TLC Scanner II/HP computer serie 200

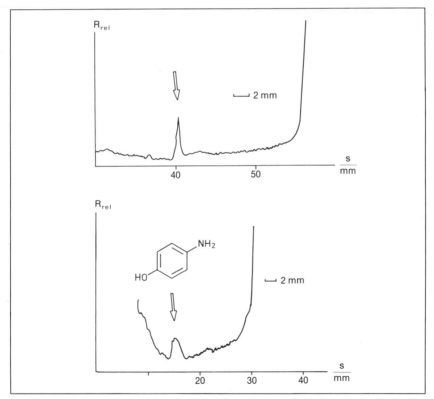

Fig. 9: TLC of 4-aminophenol as degradation product of acetaminophen
A: HPTLC   B: TLC-plates with concentration zone   C: HPTLC with AMD

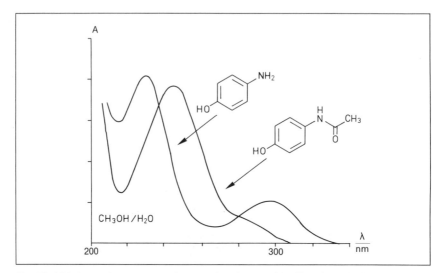

Fig. 10: UV absorption spectra of acetaminophen and its first degradation product 4-aminophenol

problem plates with concentration zones as manufactured by Merck or the automated multiple development (AMD) (10) have advantages compared to normally used TLC techniques (11).

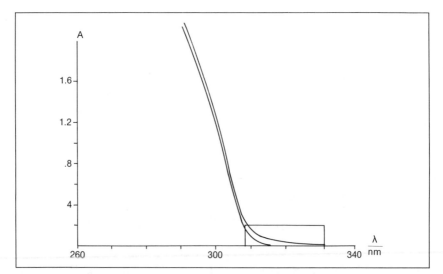

Fig. 11: UV absorption spectra of acetaminophen (20.00 mg/100 ml) (A) and acetaminophen (20.00 mg/100 ml) in presence of 4-aminophenol (0.403 mg/100 ml) (B)

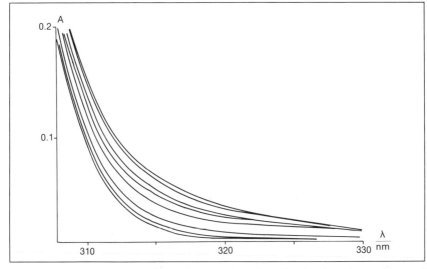

Fig. 12: Enlarged scale uv absorption spectra of acetaminophen in presence of different amounts of 4-aminophenol and different matrices

4. UV-Spectrometry

At the first glance spectrometric analyses in the uv region for stability testing seem to be an insufficient method if a limit of determination of 0.1 to 0.5% is needed. In the case of 4-aminophenol as degradation product of paracetamol the maxima of absorbance are 250 nm resp. 235 and 301 nm. From fig. 10 it is evident that only the small absorption peak of 4-aminophenol can be used if possible.

The problems arizing in stability testing are seen from fig. 11 where the spectra of pure paracetamol and paracetamol with 2% 4-aminophenol are compared. There are slight differences at the higher wavelength region depending on the concentration of 4-aminophenol (fig. 12).

UV spectrometric analyses are proposed using the following technique of data evaluation (12): First difference spectra are generated subtracting the spectrum of pure paracetamol (fig. 13 A). In order to eliminate irregular absorption caused by the matrix of the drug formulation the spectra are normalized to zero absorptivity at 340 nm (fig. 13 B). There is only the assumption of linear background absorption between 310 and 340 nm.

For quantitative analyses absorption of the normalized difference spectra at 315 nm is used. Using synthetic mixtures of 4-aminophenol (0.2 mp to 2%) and paracetamol a sufficient accuracy and precision was obtained. The calibration line with its confidence interval is presented in fig. 14. Somewhat better results are obtained using the slope of the difference spectra between 310 and 320 nm calculated by linear regression.

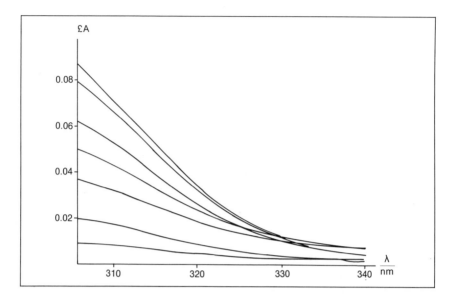

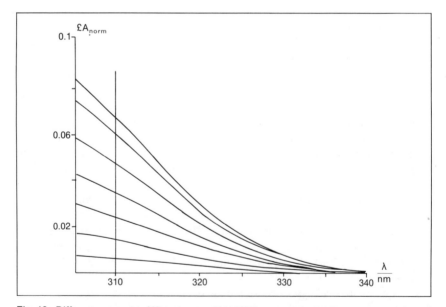

Fig. 13: Difference spectra (A) and normalized difference spectra (B) of 4-aminophenol

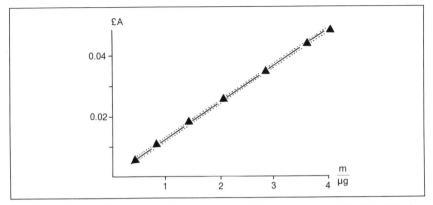

Fig. 14: Calibration line and confidence intervall of the uv spectrometric determination of 4-aminophenol in acetaminophen

This proposed method can be used easily in stress stability testing of acetamino-phen formulations as solutions or syrupe where the nonstressed formulation is used as standard for the difference spectra. In other cases the content of non degradated acetaminophen has to be determined for instance by uv spectrometry after dilution. Error analysis had been done (12) with the result that an error of 2% in the undegradated acetaminophen may be neglected in determination of 4-aminophenol. This disadvantage is overcome by another method of data evaluation using convolution or cross correlation techniques (13). For convolution orthogonal polynomials of second order centred at 302 nm with 21 points are used. The convolution technique is described in (5). Cross correlation is done in the spectral range between 320 and 300 or 320 nm.

5. Voltammetry

Many assay methods for acetaminophenol are reported in the literature (3), (4). The classical paper of Shearer and coworkers (14) on voltammetric determination of acetaminophen using a glassy carbon electrode has to correct the baseline if p-aminophenol is present. This is overcome by the used linear direct current voltammetry. Differential pulse voltammetry as used by Munson (15) for determin-ation of acetaminophen in plasma has the advantages of higher sensitivity and of separating the peaks of p-aminophenol and acetaminophen and therefore may be used for stability testing of this drug (16). Voltammetry of acetaminophen and its metabolites with electrode reactions as main topic was reported by Kissinger (17).

There are two main but typical problems in voltammetry at solid electrodes: reproducibility of measured curves and baselines and otherwise changes in the

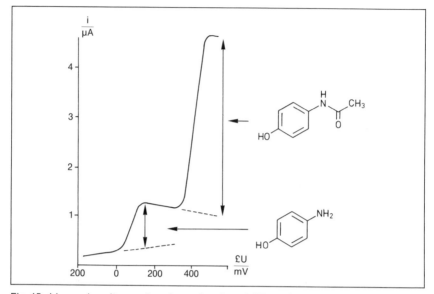

Fig. 15: Linear dc voltammetry of p-aminophenol (25 ppm) in presence of acetaminophen (100 ppm) (14)

electrode surface caused by the reaction products of the determination. Different scans in the same solution will lead to a decrease in peakhight and a change of the peak potential to more positive voltages (fig. 15). The magnitude of this effect is depending on the concentration of analyte. At low concentrations it becomes negligible. But also at lower concentrations the electrode surface will be changed and the electrode has to be repolished and reconditioned.

Surface effects from these procedures have a high influence on the shape of baseline and the current efficiency. From these items it is evident that after each repolishing procedure calibration has to be renewed to overcome the changed sensitivity (fig. 18).

6. Titration procedures

Most analysts believe that titration procedures does not work in drug stability testing. The reason should be low selectivity and low sensitivity and lack of precision as microprocedure. If we look at the choosen example of determination of 4-aminophenol at levels below 1% in presence of acetaminophen all assumptions are not valid. Contrary to acetaminophen the hydrolysis product aminophenol is very easily oxidized or may be titrated by sodium nitrite to form an aromatic diazonium salt. Both titration procedures should be selective. While there are problems in redox

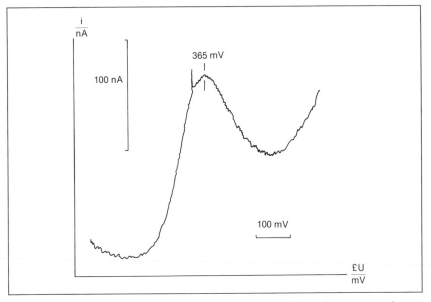

Fig. 16: Differential pulse voltametry of p-aminophenol (0.6 ppm) presence of acetaminophen (16)

titrations – acetaminophen is oxidized even by iodine – no problems are arising in nitritometric determination using voltammetric determination of the endpoint. Using sodium nitrite (c = 0.01 mol/l) one milliliter of the reagent solution is equivalent to 1.09 mg 4-aminophenol. Taking an aliquot of about 200 mg acetaminophen a degradation of 0.5% only 1 ml sodium nitrite solution is needed to reach the equivalence point. Computer controlled titration systems (18), (19) using bivoltammetric endpoint determination will have a precision of about 1% of the reagent volume and are able to handle reagent volumes down to 0.5 ml with this precision. The titration curves are evaluated by the tangent-method (fig. 19), acetaminophen does not interfere (20).

7. Conclusions

Using stability testing of acetaminophen a widely used analgesic drug the application of different analytical procedures are reported in order to amphesize that not only commonly used HPLC procedures with uv detection are the state of art. A good practising analyst does not use only one method and adopt this method to all his problems. There are more than 250 papers in the literature for derivatization of barbituric acids to more volatile compounds applicable to gaschromatography at

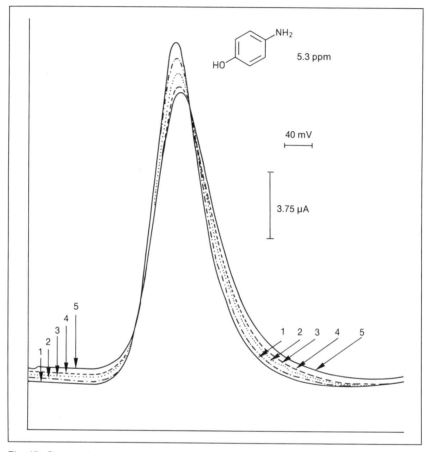

Fig. 17: Successive scans of p-aminophenol (5.3 ppm) demonstrating changes in the surface of electrode by the oxidized analyte

such levels of concentrations where other methods as HPLC, TLC are more sufficient, but a lot of these papers had not been necessary if analysts had looked to other analytical procedures. HPLC is a trend, is a must and is a high prestige method at this time and a lot of people believe to HPLC as a bible but are not looking, how many compounds are eluting in the one peak used for determination of a special compound. Good laboratory practise in the real meaning of this often used term is not only to do statistics on the special problem as it is often understood. More, it is the research to find out the most selective, the most sensitive and the most accurate method out of the whole field of analytical procedures for the given special problem. From this reason different analytical procedures has been discussed to show up that for instance spectrometric methods or simple titrations have not to be forgotten besides socalled modern instrumental methods.

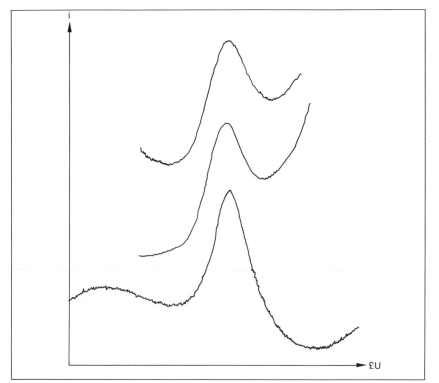

Fig. 18: Peaks in voltammetry of p-aminophenol (about 0.5 to 0.6 ppm) at the same electrode after repolishing and reconditioning

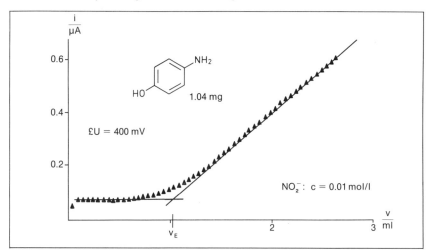

Fig. 19: Titration of 4-aminophenol with NO_2^--solution and amperometric endpoint-determination (20)

Acknowledgement

All experimental research was especially elaborated for this paper by W. Mück (HPLC with PAD and ECD), M. Herboth (TLC), W. Bender (UV spectrometry), B. Reyer and U. Kurzknabe (potentiometric titrations), M. Lorz (amperometric titrations) and F.J. Placke and B. Mümmler (voltammetry) as a round robin test or competition of analytical procedures. The research was sponsored by Deutsche Forschungsgemeinschaft, Bundesgesundheitsamt Berlin and Fonds der Chemischen Industrie.

References

(1) S. Ebel, R. Bender, M. Mück and A. Werner-Busse: Fresenius Z. Anal. Chem. *320*, 671 (1985).
(2) A. Werner-Busse: Thesis Würzburg 1985.
(3) J.E. Fairbrother in K. Florey (Edit.): Analytical Profiles of Drug Substances *3*, 1 (1974), Academic Press New York and London.
(4) H.A. El-Obeid and A.A. Al-Badr in K. Florey (Edit.): *14*, 551 (1985).
(5) A.M. Wahbi, S. Ebel and U. Steffens: Fresenius Z. Anal. Chem. *273*, 183 (1975).
(6) M. Goto, Y. Koyanagy and D. Ishii: J. Chromatogr. *208*, 261–68 (1981).
(7) J.M. Wilson, J.T. Slattery, A.J. Forth and S.D. Nelson: J. Chromatogr. *227*, 453–62 (1982).
(8) S. Ebel and W. Mück: to be published.
(9) W. Mück, H. Völter and W. Weiss: unpublished results.
(10) K. Burger: Fresenius Z. Anal. Chem. *318*, 228 (1984).
(11) S. Ebel and M. Herboth: to be published.
(12) S. Ebel and R. Bender: unpublished results.
(13) S. Ebel, R. Bender and W. Mück: to be published.
(14) C.M. Shearer, K. Christenson, A. Mukkerji and G.J. Papariello: J. Pharm. Sci. *61*, 1627–30 (1972).
(15) J.W. Munson and H. Abdine: J. Pharm. Sci. *67*, 1775–76 (1978).
(16) S. Ebel, P. Kiechle, B. Mümmler and F.J. Placke: to be published.
(17) D.J. Miner, J.R. Rice, R.M. Riggin and P.T. Kissinger: Anal. Chem. *53*, 2258–63 (1981).
(18) S. Ebel, J. Hocke and B. Reyer: Fresenius Z. Anal. Chem. *308*, 437 (1981).
(19) S. Ebel, M. Lorz and B. Reyer: to be published.
(20) S. Ebel and M. Lorz: unpublished results.

XV. Analytical procedures for stability testing of phytopharmaka and pharmaceutical products derived from natural compounds

G. Harnischfeger, Schaper & Brümmer, D-Salzgitter

1. Introduction

The term "phytopharmakon" is defined in a variety of ways to characterize a multitude of pharmaceutical preparations found mostly in the OTC section of pharmacies and drugstores. For the purpose of this article the following definition for this type of drug is used:

"A phytopharmakon constitutes a therapeutic agent or pharmaceutical speciality (i. e. commercial package of a formulated drug) intended for classical, conventional medical treatment. Its active ingredients are derived from herbal and animal raw materials".

The properties given in table 1 define the phytopharmakon even further and set definite limitations for its use.

The definition as given above excludes all drugs used in alternative therapeutic concepts such as homeopathy, anthroposophy and phytotherapy. This is important since the requirements for a meaningful stability test have to be derived from a pharmacologic and therapeutic consensus about the intended use of the drug in question.

All phytopharmaka in the aforementioned sense are required by the Drug Act of the Fed. Rep. of Germany from 1976 (2. AMG) to be manufactured in a proven and documented quality. This includes a documented proof for sufficient stability. A peculiarity of the Drug Act of the Fed. Rep. of Germany constitutes the requirement that not only prescription medicines but also drugs found in the OTC section and therefore intended for self-medication have to comply fully with the laid down

Table 1: Dr. Götz Harnischfeger

Definition of Phytopharmakon	
Active ingredients:	● total extracts or isolated components of a drug/plant
	● chemically defined single active component from a drug/plant as long as it is used in *OTC* medicines
Proprietary drug:	● approved
	● ethical
	● no predominantly homoeopathic declaration

standards of pharmaceutical quality. For those pharmaceutical specialities which were already on the market at the time of introduction of the new Drug Act in 1976, the documented proof has to be provided by December 31st, 1989.

The fulfillment of the legal requirements for quality poses a problem, since in phytopharmaka the medically active component is in most cases one or more extracts, which are in themselves a multi-component mixture as a rule. An extract contains besides biologically active compounds in various concentrations components which are only supportive in the sense that they e. g. facilitate resorption, and also components which are inactive and constitute ballast. In addition the therapeutic effect is in many cases expressed in rather general terms and cannot be reduced to known components in the respective extracts conforming to a strict pharmacological dose-response mechanism. Fundamental research covering the pharmacological and phytochemical basis is lacking to a large extent, which makes the situation of the already complex problem of multi-component mixtures even more difficult, especially since a methodical development of the field was largely neglected. In spite of these extraordinary obstacles it is possible to standardize many phytopharmaka in regard to constant and reliable quality. Such standardization is a basic requirement for a scientifically sound determination of stability.

Presently, the efforts of the relevant industry in the Fed. Rep. of Germany are mainly concerned with establishing the stability of specialities already available in the market. That means that the manufacturer has to give evidence of sufficient stability for *already existing* formulations and recipes. Changes which are suggested from the results of such stability tests cannot easily be put into effect since the composition of the speciality, at least in its active ingredients, has to be preserved. This situation of phytopharmaceuticals is dealt with primarily in this contribution. For a newly developed speciality a simplification of the outlined procedures will in many cases suffice.

2. General requirements

The legal requirement for approval of a pharmaceutical speciality includes the documentation of sufficient stability. Stability is in this case defined as constant quality over a reasonable period of time in respect to galenic, physical, chemical, biological and micro-biological parameters. In more simple terms, it means that the specifications of the quality control for the manufactured product have to be continuously met during this period of time. The pharmaceutical product is considered stable as long as the content of every single active ingredient does not fall short of 90% of the declared value and as long as probable degradation-products are non-toxic.

Phytopharmaka are in this regard nothing special and have to fulfill the aforementioned requirements as well. The analytical peculiarities inherent in this group of drugs require, however, a more differentiated approach. In planning a stability test the following, additional considerations have to be included:

- The specifications for the final control in manufacturing and those of the stability test can differ due to stability surcharges.
- The intended analytical methods have to be specific for the evaluation of stability, e. g. they have to allow for a determination of degradation-products.
- Stress testing is, as a rule, inadequate.
- Cloudiness and slight sedimentation are the rule rather than the exception for liquid forms of phytopharmaka. One has, therefore, to examine if this does or does not involve a loss of active principles.
- The rule of thumb, that the most instable component determines the stability, has to be restricted in a first approximation to components of primary importance for the medical indication of the speciality in question. The quantitative determination should, therefore, be concerned primarily with these components.
- Other, less important, components e. g. those added for galenical reasons should only be examined in a qualitative manner (fingerprint-TLC). Into this category should be counted e. g. herbal drugs added as colouring or flavouring additives in tea mixtures.

In regard to physical and micro-biological stability no differing approach is required for phytopharmaka compared with normal prescription drugs. The relevant published literature covers adequately this section of stability testing.

3. Procedure for the planning of a stability test

Considerations of time and technical expenditure render it in general impossible to include *all* components of an extract or a speciality made thereof in the investigation. This is due to the multitude of ingredients. The investigation has to be restricted to the consideration of selected, critical components.

Therefore, as a first step, a classification of components with regard to relevance has to be made. This is, however, only possible if an exact definition of the medical indication of the speciality is available. The latter is by no means self-evident for most OTC products.

Fig. 1 gives the flow-chart of the sequence of necessary information and decisions which form the background for the methodical outlay of a stability study. They are detailed in the following.

Most important, the medical indication of the speciality to be tested has to be clearly defined. This definition encompasses the affliction which has to be treated, the therapeutic aim and the dosage necessary to achieve it. The definitions have to provide as much detail as possible. It is e.g. inadequate to define an urologic preparation as useful "for inflammation and irritation of the urinary passages" without any further specification as "antibacterial and spasmolytically active". The lattter addition allows to select from the multitude of plant components and pharmacological models available for testing those with first relevance. The therapeutic aim can be derived from this as: "diminishing the germ count in the urine and elimination of bacteriuria, inhibition of an ascension of germs into the kidney, reduction of micturition difficulties and pressure sensivity of the region of the bladder". The intended therapeutic period and dosage has also to be defined e.g. 20 days for a dosage of e.g. 3×5 ml daily. This allows to specify relevant components even further due to considerations of quantity and time.

After a selection of medically relevant components has been achieved, the testing methodology and analytical techniques have to be worked out with special regard to qualitative and quantitative accuracy. No possible deviation should go undetected and must be clearly identifiable. The analytical procedures can be chemical, physical or biological in nature, great emphasis has to be placed on simple and easy techniques.

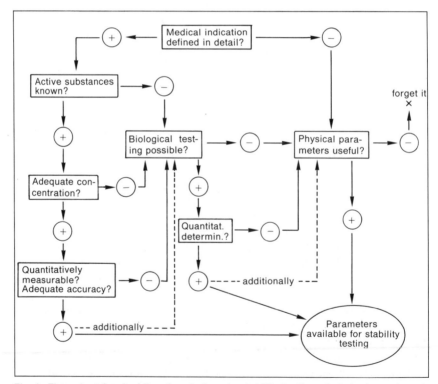

Fig. 1: Flow-chart for deciding the strategy in stability testing of phytopharmaka

Table 2: Prerequisite information required for the planning of stability testing of phytopharmaka

---

1. Medical indication of the drug speciality
   - specified symptomatology of the disease to be treated
   - therapeutical aim and target organ
   - recommended dosage

2. Ingredient substances known to be active in relation to items stated in 1
   - concentration in the drug speciality
   - qualitative/quantitative analytic methods
   - possible changes during storage
     (Redox reactions, rearrangements, hydrolysis etc.)
   - factors influencing the above alterations
     (pH, ionic strength, solvent, temperature etc.)

3. Galenical formulation
   - susceptibility to phase separation, precipitation, turbidity
   - susceptibility to micro-organisms
   - factors influencing the items stated in 2.

The medical use of many of the presently available phytopharmaka is based in folk medicine. The active ingredients are insufficiently known; or, known active ingredients are only part of active complexes in which they are contained in insufficient concentration. Especially in such cases one has to adapt to a biological determination of activity. Unfortunately, only a limited amount of quantitative biological techniques are available. Their results are as a rule susceptible to large deviations and they require personnel experienced in animal experimentation.

If neither chemical or physico-chemical nor biological methods can be used, one has to consider if stability can be determined through general physical parameters like dry residue, density, pH etc.

If even this is not possible, then speculation reigns. For example, for tonica based on red-wine containing a low dosage of extracts from 20 to 30 herbs an exact stability test which investigates more than micro-biological quality is not possible.

The above-mentioned considerations provide a frame from which the plan for the investigation of stability can be derived. The prospective analytical procedures are narrowed in a further step using additional restraints due to technical considerations. Table II puts these in a logical sequence with those already mentioned. The technical considerations are

3.1 predictable chemical changes

If chemical structures are known for the components selected for stability testing, then possible alterations can be predicted. The analytical method which will be selected for the investigation must, as a consequence, be able to recognize these plausible reaction products. Such chemical alterations are mainly caused by the following type of reactions

3.1.1 Redox reactions;

Redox reactions occur predominantly in those pharmaceutical specialities which contain plant extracts in aqueous or non-alcoholic form. Such reactions are normally catalyzed by enzymes, such as ubiquitous phenol oxidases and peroxidases co-extracted during manufacture. The risk of instability can be greatly reduced during manufacture by testing for latent peroxidase activity and subsequent measures for its inactivation.

3.1.2 Interconversions;

Especially flavane derivatives can be altered in aqueous/alcoholic solution through acid-base catalysis. Plant extracts possess usually a pH between 2 and 4 due to co-extraction of organic plant acids, so that such interconversions are in the realm of possibility. An example is given by the conversion of isoliquiritigenine/liquiritigenine (fig. 2).

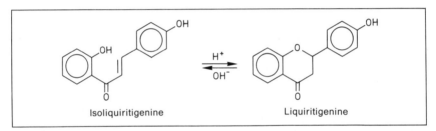

Fig. 2: Example of an acid-catalyzed conversion

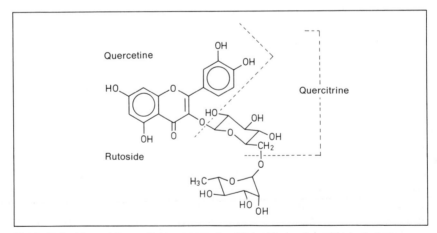

Fig. 3: Rutoside and its partial components obtainable in glycoside hydrolysis

3.1.3 Hydrolysis;

Acid catalyzed hydrolysis is one way for chemical change in many glycosides. A well-known example is rutoside (fig. 3) which is split into its various components by heat and acid pH (e.g. sterilization of an injectable solution).

3.1.4 Condensations and polymerisations;

These types of reactions play a special role if catechine and catechine-derivatives are present in the phytopharmakon (e.g. in Crataegi flos). Fig. 4 depicts the mechanism given by WEINGES et al. (1969).

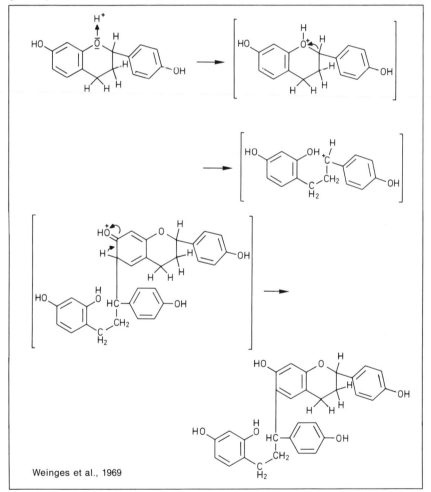

Fig. 4: Mechanism of the acid-catalyzed self-condensation of catechines

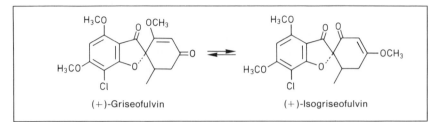

Fig. 5: Example of an isomerisation

3.1.5 Isomerisations;

This tpye of alteration is depicted in fig. 5 using griseofulvin as an example.

3.1.6 Photochemical processes;

Photochemically induced changes are quite frequent in pharmaceutical products and are found not only in the text-book example reserpine. For example, menthone in aqueous/ethanolic solution is changed by sunlight into menthocitronellal and a saturated acid (fig. 6). Similar processes, this time with free radicals as intermediates, are known for camphora (fig. 7) which is an ingredient of about 250 pharmaceutical preparations, many of those phytopharmaka, in the Fed. Rep. of Germany.

There is a number of other possibilites for chemical alterations which were not mentioned. One example is the time-dependent change of valepotriates into baldrinales where the underlying mechanism became known in the last few years with great repercussion on the stability data of preparations containing Valerianae radix.

The qualitative demonstration of the above-mentioned processes is in theory relatively simple since initially present components disappear and new ones are formed. Main emphasis has to be placed onto chromatographic fingerprint analysis. The observation of framework conditions, e.g. pH, ionic strength, density, flocculation and opacity can give additional important hints. A small degree of turbidity is, by the way, common in liquids due to the interaction of acid tannines with the alkali of the bottle material "glass". This factor does not need to be considered in evaluating the stability of the preparation.

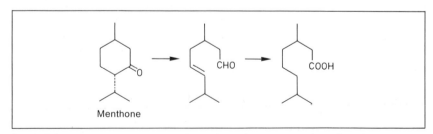

Fig. 6: Photochemical conversion of menthone in aqueous ethanolic solution

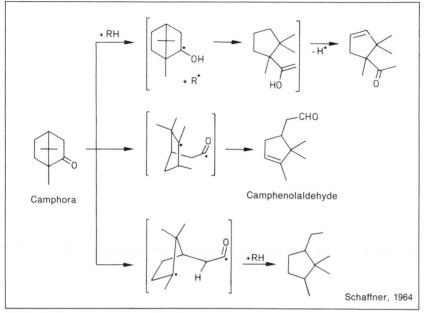

Fig. 7: Photochemical conversion of camphora

3.2 Predictable galenical changes

The stability of multi-component mixtures constitutes primarily a "lability" since the ingredients of phytopharmaka, – and that includes the auxiliary components for the galenical formulation –, are mostly in a very precarious balance with each other. This is especially true for solutions where equilibria can be very easily destroyed through physical interactions e. g. agglomerations. Flocculation and turbidity are thus almost unavoidable by-products during storage. This fact has to be kept in mind. It is especially relevant in assessing the stability of injectable solutions containing plant extracts. Turbidity and flocculation constitute not a slowly proceeding process but occur within a very narrow period of time in a very massive way. Fig. 8 illustrates this as an example for an extract containing tannines. The tannine molecules form polymers, turbidity becomes manifest and, after some more time, a complete flocculation, sedimentation and subsequent clearing of the solution take place.

Galenical incompatibilities should always be expected, especially, if several extracts are combined in the marketed phytopharmakon. The main attention has to be placed in this case onto the co-extractives and not onto the components important and selected for biological activity. This is easy to see, since during development of the pharmaceutical speciality its active ingredients are much more likely to be considered in detail. Physical and chemical interactions between co-extractives are often overlooked, but can greatly influence the stability. Fig. 9 shows such possible interactions.

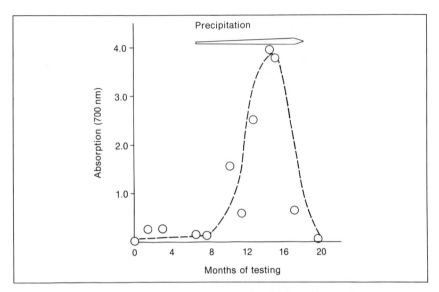

Fig. 8: Time course of turbidity and precipitation in a high-grade tannine plant extract

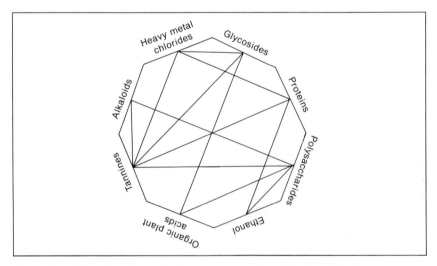

Fig. 9: Possible interactions between groups of plant ingredients and extract components

4. Technical limitations in stability testing of phytopharmaka

Besides limitations in the analytical procedures proper the main constriction is due to the fact that the multicomponent mixture "phytopharmakon" is tested using a *subjective* selection of components while interactions between other compounds of the preparation have to be practically ignored. With other words, the hypothesis of "pars pro toto" constitutes the basis for the stability test. Interactions not involving the selected ingredient-compounds can only be observed through galenical alterations during the test.

The selection and use of the "pars pro toto" principle is completely independent of the differentiation between monodrug speciality (i. e. one made from one herbal drug only) or a "combination" preparation. In the latter case things are similar but more complicated.

The "pars pro toto" principle is also the reason that methods using accelerated, e. g. stress, testing are of limited usefulness only. Stress testing is based on the assumption that the active component degrades by a kinetic of first order, which is quite improbable considering the multitude of components which influence, e. g., the stability of an extract. Therefore, long-term stability testing has to be emphasized for phytopharmaka.

The logic of stability testing is even more strained if active components for the medical indication are not known, are in doubt, or stability can only be determined through biological tests and galenical considerations. The variability of data obtained with biological methods is much greater than with data obtained through chemical analysis.

A stability evaluation which is based on physical (galenical) data alone, due to lack of suitable chemical or biological methods, can only be assigned a very low grade of credibility in respect to constant therapeutical effects and absence of unforeseen risks in the intended shelf-life. Exceptions can only be seen in preparations containing essential oils as active ingredients.

5. Methods and their limitations

Stability testing of phytopharmaka has a quantitative and a qualitative aspect of which the latter has a very high significance. In most cases, qualitative data give the only hint that alterations during storage took place.

Physico-chemical procedures encompass nowadays the bulk of analytical methods. Especially the chromatographic separation-procedures GC, HPLC and TLC are used either alone or in combination with spectrophotometry. A few examples are given and should suffice. Fig. 10 shows the separation of concentrated Melilotus-extract using TLC and cochromatography with reference substances. Fig. 11 depicts the gaschromatographical identification of 13 herbal drugs used in a

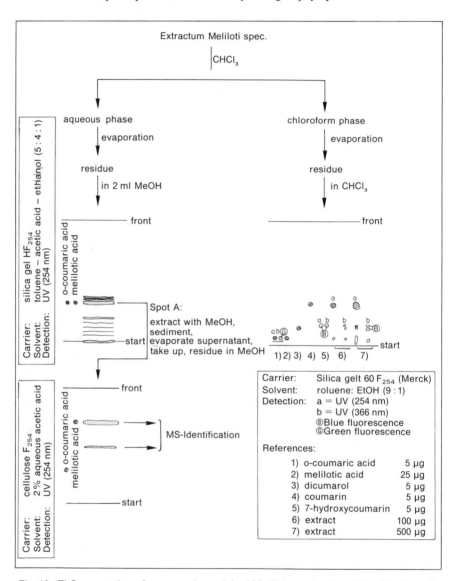

Fig. 10: TLC-separation of a coumarin-enriched Melilotus extract and identification of separated substances through cochromatography

	Spirit of carmelites	Melissae folium	Cinnamomi cortex	Caryophylli flos	Myristicae semen	Cassiae flos	Cardamomi fructus	Piperis nigri fructus	Aurantii pericarpium	Angelicae radix	Gentianae radix	Galangae rhizoma	Helenii rhizoma	Zingiberis rhizoma
Aceteugenol											●			●
Camphora		●			●									●
Borneol	●													●
Camphene												●		●
Caryophyllene											●	●	●	●
Caryophyllenoxide											●		●	●
Cineol	●	●					●							●
Citral A and B	●												●	●
Citronellal													●	●
p-Cymol					●							●		●
Eugenol		●								●	●	●		●
Geraniol	●												●	●
Humulen											●			●
Limonene						●	●							●
Linalool													●	●
Myrcene						●	●							●
Myristicine										●				●
Neral	●												●	●
Pentadecanolide					●									●
Phellandrene	●				●		●					●		●
a-Pinene					●	●	●			●		●		●
Saffrole										●				●
Terpenylacetate						●		●						●
a-Terpineol								●						●
Cinnamic aldehyde												●		●
Cinnamic acid												●		●
Zingiberene/Zingiberol	●									●				●

HANKE, 1984

Fig. 11: Multi-component speciality (Tinctura Melissae comp., Carmelitergeist) containing 13 extracts and the detection of each extract-component

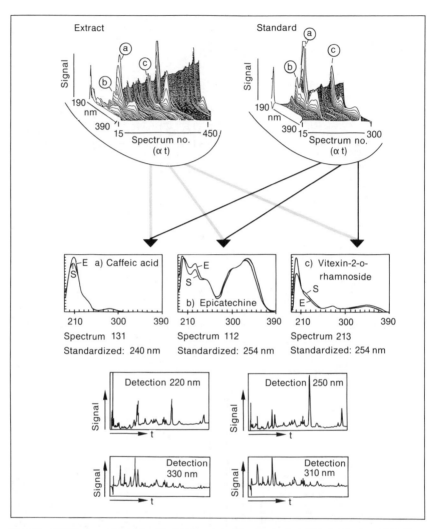

Fig. 12: HPLC separation of a Crataegus extract with on-line UV spectral registration; solvent: acetonitril – phosphoric acid – water gradient, column: Spherisorb ODS 5 µm, pump: Varian 5000; detector: photodiodearray detector Philips PU 4021; computer: Trivektor "Trilab 2000"

Application range for standard analytical methods

Analytical method	Pharmaka containing synthetic active ingredients or pure natural substances		Pharmaka with		Phytopharmaka			Homoeopathika (organic and anorganic)	
	one active ingredient only	mixture of active ingredients	minerals	organic metal complexes	one extract only	several extracts	extracts or oils with volatile substances	homoeopathics tinctures	dilutions, triturations
Volumetry	++	±	±	+	±	−	±	−	−
Photometry	++	±	+	+	+	(+)	±	±	−
Fluorometry	(+)	±	−	−	−	−	−	−	−
DC/HPTLC Densiometry	++	++	+	+	++	+	++	++	+
GC (+MS)	(+)	(++)	−	−	(+)	(+)	+	(++)	(++)
HPLC	+	++	+	+	++	++	+	++	++
¹H-NMR	++	−	−	−	−	−	(±)	−	−
¹³C-NMR	++	(−)	−	+	−	−	−	−	−
MS	++	−	−	−	−	−	−	−	−
IR	+	±	−	++	−	−	−	−	−
UV/VIS	+	−	−	++	−	−	−	−	−
AAS	−	−	++	++	−	−	−	++	+

++ = well-suited, + = suited, ± = suited but limited, − = not suited, ( ) = the limitation of analytical method to be used and the physico-chemical properties of the substances have to be taken into consideration.

TITTEL, 1984

Fig. 13: Field of application for standard analytical methods

"Tinctura melissae comp." The above-mentioned methods are primarily separating procedures, but they allow also the selection of those ingredients to be quantitatively measured. Especially the method of HPLC has been combined with on-line coupling of photometry and fast computing for correcting distortions in the spectra and quantitative measuring of single peaks. An example is given in fig. 12.

The possible range of instrumental analysis and their usefulness in the analysis of phytopharmaka is tabulated in fig. 13.

6. Combination products

Before investigating combinations (i.e. products manufactured from various combined drugs or extracts), one has to assess if the active substances selected from the investigation are present in only one or in several of the herbal drugs used, and if the quantitative analysis method to be chosen determines selectively compounds or groups of substances only (table 3). If groups of substances are determined in analysis, one has to be aware of the fact that interconversions within such groups, e. g. within the flavonoids, cannot be detected.

With herbal teas and preparations made directly out of the cut drug material, one has to consider that the content given in the pharmacopeia is a minimum value from which the actual value cannot fall short.

In practice, it is in many cases impossible to directly test quantitatively the stability behaviour of multi-component preparations. Under those circumstances, there is a *strictly empirical* way out, i.e. every single extract is tested in combination with the auxiliary substances used for the final product. The stability of that active extract

Table 3

Quantitative content of flavone glycosides in drugs					
Drug	Vitexin-2''-O-rhamnosid	Vitexin	Rutin	Hyperosid	Quercitrin
Arnicae mont. flos	–	ST	–	–	0,08
Betulae folium	–	ST	–	0,53	0,09
Crataegi folium c. flore	0,53	0,02	0,17	0,28	ST
Crataegi flos	0,21	0,014	0,16	0,69	ST
Crataegi folium	0,55	0,03	0,29	0,19	ST
Heterothecae flos	–	–	0,3	0,22	ST
Passiflorae herba	–	0,02	0,27	0,02	ST
Tiliae flos	–	–	–	0,25	0,25

The above figures show the percentage values for the individual drugs; ST = standard

STUMPF, 1985

with the lowest shelf-like determines the storage-span of the entire preparation. It has to be made sure, however, that interactions between the various extracts are unlikely to occur. Such interactions can be easily detected through physical data (e. g. change in pH) and sensory analysis.

Sensory analysis has not been reported in stability testing of pharmaceutical products. It should, however, be possible to obtain useful results also in combination preparations, if the methods are exactly defined. Such determinations are state of the art in food technology. Only the determination of the bitter principle plays a role in pharmacy.

7. Examples

The necessary data on stability can be obtained, in most cases, with the standard analytical methods available in an industrial laboratory. This will be explained in the following examples.

7.1 Combination speciality: purified plant extract, standardized onto the active substance coumarin plus rutoside as second active ingredient; soft gelatine-capsule:

The stability testing involves in this case two substances which can be sufficiently separated using HPLC. Co-extractives like o-coumaric acid, melilotic acid etc. are

Preparation:

V 1004

Active substances: Extr. Melilot. stand. containing coumarin, rutoside;

Soft-gelatine capsule

Storage conditions: Storage for 5 years at room temperature

contents in %	Coumarin	Rutin
at production	98.4 ± 5.5	100.9 ± 5.5
after 5 years	97.6 ± 4.0 84.7% thereof in the capsule filling, 13.1% in the gelatine capsule itself	94.8 ± 4.2

Weight:	at production	437 ± 5
	after 5 years	445 ± 4
Dissolution (min.):	at production	8.8 ± 1.7
	after 5 years	14.3 ± 0.7

Fig. 14: Results of stability testing for a phytopharmakon composed of two active substances.

under 10% of the coumarin content and can, therefore, be neglected. This is argued from the natural concentration gradient in the plant (about 1 to 5) and the selective extraction.

Fig. 14 shows the stability data. Because of low vapour-pressure part of the coumarin diffuses into the gelatine-capsule itself which, however, is not a negative mark since the gelatine-capsule is also digested.

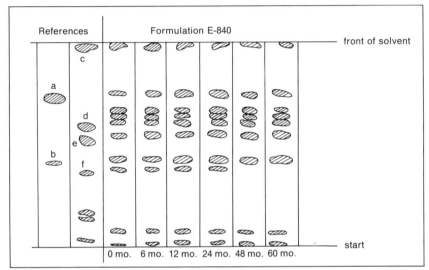

Fig. 15: Qualitative (TLC) determination of stability of a Crataegus extract

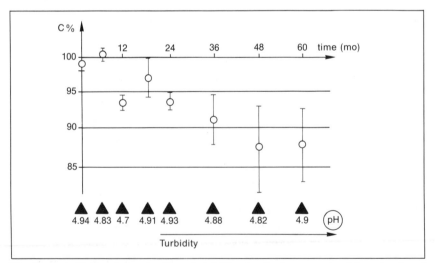

Fig. 16: Quantitative determination of stability of a Crataegus extract (gravimetry of condens. flavanes)

Table 4: Stability data of a flavonoid containing liquid

Peak	\(mg flavonoids/100 ml\)					
	0 months	6 months	12 months	24 months	36 months	48 months
1	6.2	6.7	6.5	6.2	6.15	6.1
2	16.22	15.4	15.9	15.2	14.9	15.0
3	24.0	29.4	22.3	22.0	21.9	20.2
4	4.21	4.3	4.15	4.1	3.9	3.5
5	4.41	3.7	3.7	3.5	2.5	2.1
6–13*	94.26	87.2	86.55	84.6	84.15	83.6
1–13	149.3	140.7	139.1	133.6	135.5	130.5
%	100	94.2	93.2	90.82	89.4	87.4

* Peaks 6–13 were measured separately, the results are given as a sum for technical resons only.

STUMPF, 1985

7.2 Mono-extract preparation: a liquid containing Crataegi extractum. Parameter for standardization and stability testing is the content of flavane derivatives, the main components for the pharmacological activity.

Stability testing has to use two approaches. Quantitatively the flavanes can be determined only as a group by gravimetry. The investigation for alterations and decomposition of these substances can be performed using a qualitative comparison of chromatograms. Fig. 15 and 16 show that no alterations take place during the time span of 60 months. The slow decrease in overall contents is probably due to agglomeration and subsequent sedimentation.

Similar data have been published by STUMPF (1985) for a flavanoid containing liquid (mono-preparation); see table 4.

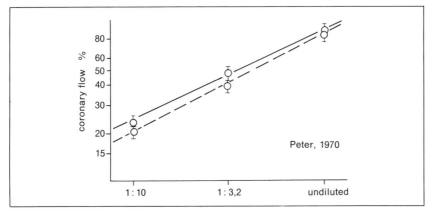

Fig. 17: Dose-effect-correlation of coronary flow in the guinea pig-Langendorff-Heart-Method (n = 26) of a freshly-prepared drug (−) and after a time span of 36 months

7.3 Biological determination of stability; injectable solution from Crataegus; determination of pharmacological activity using the guinea pig-Langendorff-Heart-Method.

PETER (1970) published values (fig. 17) which show an excellent long-term stability of the preparation in respect to its pharmacological activity.

7.4 Biological determination of stability; injectable solution with extracts from Echyrochline and Eupatorium; determination of the pharmacological effect on the immune system by evaluating the shift in the relation of leucocyte sub-populations in regard to each other.

The result given by PETER (1970) shows that the activity remains unchanged after 3 years of storage (fig. 18).

7.5 Enzymatic determination of stability of an "historic" formulation: Mixtura Pepsini:

The method for testing is given in the German pharmacopeia (DAB 6) and involves the digestion of eggwhite by pepsin. Fig. 19 shows the curve published by RICHTER (1976). The low stability of the formulation can easily be discerned. A low galenical stability, empirically found, can also be presumed from the required labelling, i. e. "shake before use". The suggested size of the formulation (200 ml) and the dosage of "3 times daily 1 tablespoon" is therefore not warranted.

Galenical not chemical stability can also be the determining factor for the shelf-life of phytopharmaka. This is demonstrated in example 6.

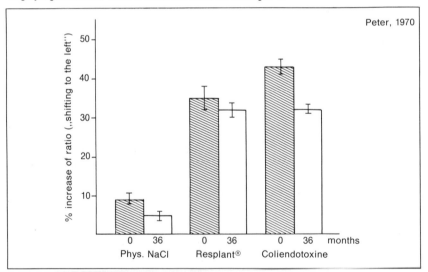

Fig. 18: "Shifting to the left" (increase in ploymorphonuclear and rod-shaped lymphocytes in the lymphocyte population) after administration of a freshly-prepared and a 36 months old immunostimulating phytopharmakon

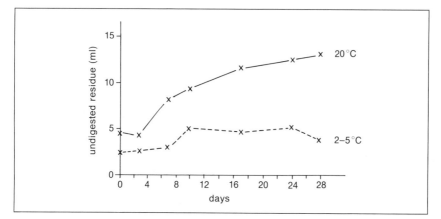

Fig. 19: Stability determination of the formulation "Mixtura Pepsini" measuring non-converted substrate

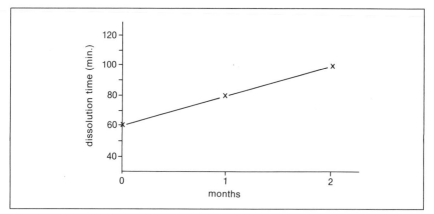

Fig. 20: Stability of Pilulae laxantes using their disintegration in vitro

7.6 Laxative pills

According to the pharmacopeia the disintegration in vitro is not allowed to exceed 60 minutes. As shown in fig. 20, the actually measured value is under 60 minutes only in the freshly prepared formulation.

8. Final remarks

The stability testing of phytopharmaka is based on *selected* parameters of physical, chemical or biological nature. This selection, necessary for the determination of stability within a reasonable time-frame and a fixed laboratory budget is, however, also the focal point for criticism. Critique is voiced particularly by scientific purists, which require an investigation of each and every component of the preparation and who are quick to point out, – in case a pragmatic solution is given –, the absence of what they consider important data. Mostly, such arguments are a camouflage for altruistic motives such as a general refusal to accept phytopharmaka as valid drugs and/or reasons stemming from market considerations. There are plenty of examples of this way of thinking to be found in the decisions of evaluation boards; fortunately, at least for us Germans, not with the BGA.

Right now, the discussion concerning use and effectiveness of medical drugs, especially phytopharmaka, has evolved into dimensions reminiscent of the theological warfare of the 16th century.

As a consequence, the defense of a scientific and technical pragmatism is presently especially tiresome and often of a disappointing futility.

There remains the hope that common sense does not get lost in the turmoil, at least not among the specialists. The contribution of this article should be understood in this way.

References

G. Ciamician, P. Silber: Chemische Lichtwirkungen XI. Ber. Dtsch. Chem. Ges. *40*, 2415, 1907

G. Hanke: Qualität pflanzlicher Arzneimittel Wiss. Verlagsges., Stuttgart 1984

H. Peter: Über die pharmakologische Qualitätsprüfung phytotherapeutischer Injektionslösungen. Phys. Med. Rehab. 1970 (4), 71–73

J. Richter: Storage problems associated with the control of medicines. pg 65–82 in Deasy, Timoney eds: The quality control of medicines, Elsevier, Amsterdam 1976

K. Schaffner: Phytochemische Umwandlung ausgewählter Naturstoffe. Fortschr. Chem. Org. Naturstoffe *22*, 1–114, 1964

T.R. Seshadri: Interconversions of flavonoid components. pg 156–196 in T.A. Geissman ed.: The chemistry of flavonoid compounds, Pergamon Press, Oxford 1962

H. Stumpf: Qualitätssicherung von Endprodukten und Fertigarzneimitteln, die Extrakte enthalten. pg 104–119 in: G. Harnischfeger ed.: Qualitätskontrolle von Phytopharmaka, Thieme, Stuttgart 1985

G. Tittel: Qualitätskontrolle in der Pharmazie, Kriterien für die Auswahl von Analysenverfahren für Arzneimitteluntersuchungen. Pharm. Ind., Sonderheft, 1984

R. Weinges, W. Bähr, W. Ebert, K. Göritz, H.D. Marx: Konstitution, Entstehung und Bedeutung der Flavonoid Gerbstoffe. Fortschr. Chem. Org. Naturstoffe *27*, 158–218, 1969

XVI. Stability Testing During Development

K. Krummen, SANDOZ LTD., Basle, Switzerland

1. Introduction

The person responsible for stability testing in a pharmaceutical firm engaged in research which operates worldwide finds himself confronted by a series of demands which are in part contradictory. I am one of these persons and would like to discuss these demands in what may perhaps be a somewhat overdrawn manner.

1.1 To ensure the quality of a product which has been stored (for clinical trials and for sale) he must determine which stability tests are necessary and practical and he must see to it that such tests are carried out.

1.2 He must have complete stability data from a sufficient number of batches in the market packaging covering as much of the postulated shelf-life as possible. He should take into consideration the various national regulations and recommendations which have not been standardized, with respect to test conditions and testing sequence, for instance, and he should keep abreast of the issuance of new regulations in interested countries.

1.3 In the interest of keeping costs to a minimum (and who is not talking about that today in the health field) he wants to avoid tests which, based on his experience, are only good as "fillers" in the registration dossier but contribute nothing to it scientifically.

1.4 As quickly as possible (within days or weeks) he is expected to predict whether a new formulation will have a shelf-life of 2, 3 or 5 years.

Clearly, it is difficult to reconcile all of this. Some of these problems which arise during stability testing in development will be discussed here. A pragmatic basis for this discussion will be chosen. It cannot be offered anything spectacular or new – today's laws of chemical kinetics are the same as those of years ago. What has changed (increased!) in recent years is the number of tests which are considered necessary to establish stability. Also, in addition to the classical chemical stability, other quality characteristics have gained importance, for example, dissolution rate, preservation and interaction with new packaging materials.

The work-up of stability data for a new medication is an evolutionary process. It

- Preformulation
  - Drug substance reactivities
  - Excipient Compatibility
  - Stab. of Toxicol. Supplies
- Formulation Development
  - Formulation Comparison
  - Stab. of Clinical Supplies
- Stability of Proposed Product

Fig. 1: Stability Studies during development

begins in the early developmental phase and continues through stability monitoring (follow-up stability) of the marketed product. With respect to the course stability testing and especially the test procedures follow, differences exist from firm to firm, from active ingredient to active ingredient and from dosage form to dosage form. Elements can be found, however, which are common to every stability test. A good overview is given in the article "Stability Concepts" by the PMA (Pharmaceutical Manufacturers Association) working group (1).

For a new active ingredient (new single chemical entity), and that is what we want to talk about here, the following phases can be differentiated which proceed together or consecutively (fig. 1) (1). In the preformulation phase, the reaction possibilities of the pure active ingredient with moisture, air, heat, etc. are investigated, which usually includes compatibility testing with excipients. The stability of samples for animal trials (e. g. feed mixtures) must be monitored. During formulation development the most stable variant or variants are chosen on the basis of results from stress tests and then subjected to long-term stability testing. The stability of batches which will be clinically tested must also be monitored. As these phases proceed our knowledge about the stability continually increases. Important synergetic effects come into play: experience with the pure active ingredient can be applied to dosage forms and experience with one dosage form can be applied to other dosage forms.

Considering the time which is available to me, I will confine my discussion to a few typical examples from individual phases.

2. Drug substance reactivities

The following tests are performed with the drug substance:

- drug substance in dry and moist environments.
- solutions or suspensions in buffer solutions pH 2–9 and in various solvents. Conditions are room temperature and 50 °C up to 4 weeks.
- sensitivity to light.

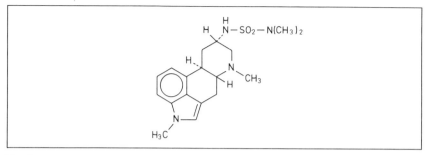

Fig. 2

Appearance and chemical degradation are evaluated; semiquantitative thin-layer chromatography suffices for this.

The active ingredient CU 32-085 was chosen as an example, a methylergoline sulphamide (fig. 2).

It was found that the drug substance only becomes discolored at 50 °C without any detectable degradation and that it is sensitive to light. When in solution or suspension in the acidic range it is unstable and sensitive to light. These investigations were supplemented by targeted degradation tests with various chemical agents which revealed the reaction possibilities shown in fig. 3. The most important degradation reaction proved to be the oxidation of the pyrol ring and positions 4 and 6. The sulphamide hydrolysis plays only a minor roll in comparison.

3. Excipient compatibility

Next the drug substance is usually examined for compatibility with common excipients. The most common procedure is storing binary mixtures of the drug substance with selected excipients at increased temperature and humidity, e. g. up to 80 °C and up to 75% R. H. for up to 12 weeks (2). Appearance and active ingredient content and decomposition are then examined.

An alternative is to test the active ingredient in mixtures of several excipients. It is preferable to use a factorial design test plan according to Yates (3) for this: In this way not only the effect of single excipients are determined, but also the interaction of several excipients with the active ingredient. An example of this is given in figure 4. It is these excipients which are commonly used for manufacturing tablets by granulation.

Two alternatives each for the filling material, the lubricant, the disintegrant and the binder are tested. The fifth factor is moisture. This produces 16 mixtures if one applies a shortened test plan. For the analysis it is advantageous if radioactively marked active ingredient is used.

For determination of intact content after storage, radiochromatography on TLC plates can be used. In addition, any content uniformity problems can be eliminated if

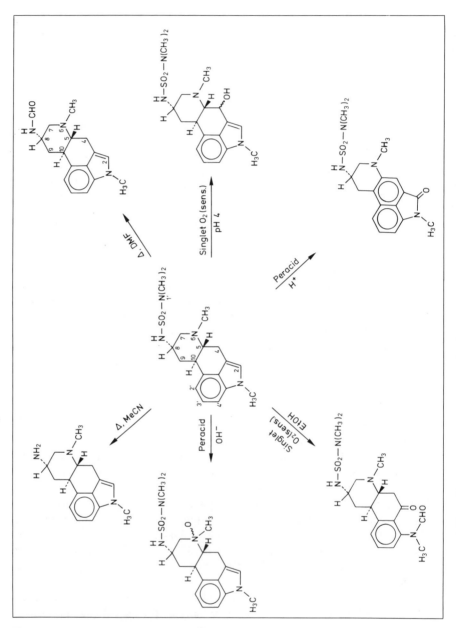

Fig. 3

Factor		Level	Composition % W/W
A	−	Lactose	75
	+	Mannitol	75
B	−	Stearic Acid	5
	+	Mg Stearate	5
C	−	Maize Starch	20
	+	Alginic Acid	20
D	−	PVP	5
	+	Hydroxypropyl-Cellulose	5
E	−	dry	
	+	70% r.H.	

Fig. 4: Factorial design for wet granulation

the radioactivity of the entire sample is measured along with the intact active ingredient on the TLC plate. For the active ingredient CU 32-085, the mixtures were stored for 8 weeks at room temperature and 50 °C. No incompatibility was shown except with stearic acid, which should be replaced by magnesium stearate. Moisture had a very negative effect.

Testing of excipient mixtures only roughly approximates the conditions in a pressed tablet; therefore, the results must be carefully interpreted. The mixture proportions greatly influence the test results. In the example in fig. 4, the amounts of stearic acid and magnesium stearate in the mixture are relatively high in order to clearly detect any interaction with these excipients which are known to be critical. In evaluating the results, this must be taken into consideration. Other critical parameters are the thoroughness of mixing and the particle size of the mixture components; they determine the contact surface between reaction partners and, therefore, greatly influence the results.

Differential scanning calorimetry (DSC) was used as a further means of studying active ingredient-excipient mixtures. It aided in selecting excipients for the direct compressing of tablets (4).

Naturally, finished sample formulations of the preparation aimed at supply a more realistic picture of the actual stability. However, their production is significantly more costly and one runs the risk of having to make a second series of sample formulations because of a single incompatibility.

With liquid forms, often the incompatibility testing phase with individual excipients or with excipient mixtures is skipped and provisional formulations of the finished dosage form are tested directly. This way the effects of gassing and sterilization on injectables can be tested at the same time. Multi-dose containers with rubber stoppers can already be checked in this phase for adsorption of active ingredient or preservatives on the stopper.

4. Formulation comparison

In this phase, various formulations are manufactured which are compared in a stress test with respect to stability. For the example, project CU 32-085, six tablet variants were produced (fig. 5): 4 with granulation and 2 with direct tabletting. The tablets were stored for 3 months at 30°C/75% R.H., 35°C and 50°C. In addition, a light exposure test and a test in a changing climate were performed. The results for appearance, proportion of degradation products and contents of intact active ingredient are summarized in fig. 6. The column-label A is for appearance, D for degradation and C for content. An empty space means no significant change. The more densely shaded a field is, the poorer the result was. Selection has based on all 3 quality characteristics because no reliable statement could be made only on the basis, for example, of the contents of intact active ingredient due to the relatively slight reduction and the unavoidable scatter of the analysis. Direct testing of degradation products is significantly more sensitive; however, the danger exists that the results turn out better than they actually are due to an undetected incomplete extraction. The determination of intact contents serves chiefly to eliminate this error.

Variants 2 and 3 were chosen for further testing. A preliminary calculation of the shelf-life was not done because the degradation products which will be limiting could only be semi-quantitatively determined. Moreover, different degradation products formed in the different variants, which is not astounding considering the active ingredient's manifold reaction possibilities.

In some cases it is better to test the physical stability in the first step and in the second step chose the best variants with respect to chemical stability (5). This is especially so for emulsions, suspensions and ointments for which the physical stability is critical. For these forms, therefore, specific stress and test methods are applied. As an example of this, 5 methods are given in fig. 7 which were used by Ondracek et al. (6) for testing the physical stability of low-viscous O/W emulsions.

	1	2	3	4	5	6
Lactose	+	+			+	+
Lactose anh.			+			
Cellulose micr.				+		
Maize starch	+	+			+	+
Ca Sulfate				+		
Maize starch paste	+				+	+
Pharmacoat		+				
NaOH					+	
NaHCO$_3$						+
Aerosil	+	+	+	+	+	+
Mg Stearate	+	+	+	+	+	+

Fig. 5: 6 tablet variants of CU 32-085 for formulation comparison

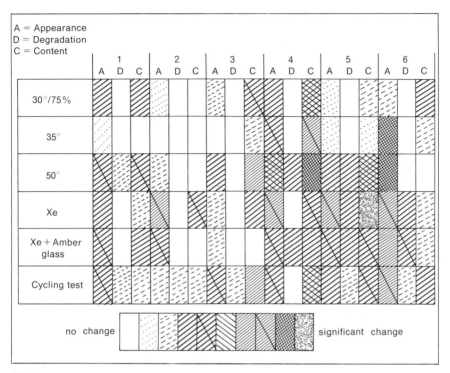

Fig. 6

The applicability of the five test procedures in forecasting stability for 8 emulsion compositions was compared. The thermostability test (appearance after 7 and 14 days at 20, 30, 40 and 50 °C) and the centrifuge test gave the best prognosis for long-term stability evaluation. Both test are, therefore, recommended for prescreening of formulations; however, other tests, e.g. microscopic examination and pH measurement, should also be applied.

Physicochemical models are often used to predict the chemical stability from stress tests, especially the Arrhenius relationship. Many examples of its application have been published. Usually homogeneous, liquid preparations are examined. A review of the literature makes an overly positive impression, however, because positive examples are more likely to be published than negative ones. Practical experience has shown though, that the Arrhenius relationship is satisfactorily fulfilled in many cases, not only for homogeneous liquid forms, but also for numerous solid and semi-solid forms. The critical points in applying the Arrhenius relationship are generally known, namely:

● the kinetics of the degradation reaction must be the same under all experimental conditions;

```
20°, 30°, 40°, 50°C
14 and 28 days
– Visual Inspection
– Centrifuge Test
– Spreading Test
– Viscosity
– Conductivity
```

Fig. 7: Methods for testing the physical stability of O/W emulsions (6)

● the data must be extremely accurate so when extrapolated to room temperature unreasonably broad confidence limits for the shelf-life do not result which would make the prediction meaningless.

At this point it will not be elaborated further on the problematics of applying of the Arrhenius relationship. There are excellent new surveys of this topic, e. g. monographs by W. Grimm and G. Schepky (7), by K. Thoma (8) and by Hartmann et al. (9) and an article by D. Kersten and B. Gröber (10). Instead two examples to stress tests in daily practice will be presented for which *physicochemical* quality characteristics are decisive.

Figure 8 shows the dissolution results for 2 different coated tablet formulations, after stress testing and after storage for several years at room temperature and 30 °C. The stress conditions were 2 months at 40 °C. The initial value is in order for both formulations. The dissolution for formulation A changes only slightly in the stress test, but for B a dramatic decrease is observed. This correlates very well with long-term results at 30 °C. At room temperature, however, formulation B is also stable.

Based on our experience, these types of stress tests with solid forms are not only suitable for testing chemical degradation, but also for examining changes in the dissolution rate and other physicochemical quality characteristics.

It is helpful if long-term experience has been had with one of the tested formulations which can so to speak build the bridge between the stress conditions and normal conditions. This way the relevance of the stress data for normal conditions is assured without mathematical models.

In many cases a reduction in the dissolution rate of tablets and coated tablets after storage runs parallel to an increase in disintegration time and sometimes in hardness. This effect has been examined in various recent papers (11–13). There is still work to be done, however, before we will be able to fully understand the causes.

The second example, fig. 9, shows the comparison of appearance for 5 tablet variants after short-term testing. Storage was for 2 months at 30 °C/65%, 30 °C/75% and 40 °C.

The 5 °C samples served as reference. The tablets, which were originally white, yellowed imperceptibly during the test – the change was practically not detectable with the naked eye. Therefore, the color difference was measured against a color standard.

Variants A and D are extremely sensitive to moisture which is recognizable from the fact that the sample stored at 30°C/75% is more discolored than the sample stored at 30°C/65% and this in turn significantly more so than the 40°C sample in tight packaging, i.e. dry, stored sample. For the other variants, B, C and E, the effects of both temperature and moisture are minor. The stress conditions were subsequently intensified: 40°C/75% without packaging was also tested. After two months, examination with the naked eye showed variants A and D bo be clearly poorer.

The relatively mild test conditions for the trial in fig. 9 sufficed, however, to clearly differentiate the samples with respect to chemical degradation. Figure 10 shows the increase in degradation products for all variants. Variant D is by far the worst, followed by A. In contrast to the change in appearance, the chemical degradation is almost identical at 30°C/65% and 35°C/75% and clearly greater than at 40°C dry.

These short-term results correspond excellently with the long-term stability results at room temperature. This is not surprising since the test conditions were not extreme stress conditions. The sensitive measurement is what is actually decisive.

In general, the experience has shown that it is advantageous to chose stress conditions which are not too drastic and then use a sensitive method of measurement so that relatively minor effects and differences are detectable. This way the application of stress results to normal conditions is more reliable. Several essential points which should be observed in planning stress tests are:

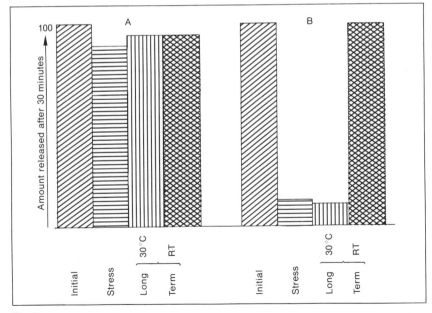

Fig. 8

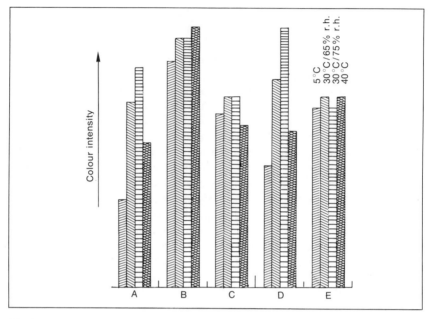

Fig. 9

- Test conditions
  - Not too exaggerated?
  - Strong enough to produce effects?
- All critical quality indications considered?
- Test method(s) sensitive enough?
- Comparison with "known" product?
- 6 or 12 months results at RT awaited?

The test conditions should not be exaggerated but still strong enough to provoke measurable effects. All quality characteristics which are critical for the shelf-life should be taken into account.

The test methods must be meaningful and sensitive, e.g. dissolution should be measured after 15 minutes instead of after 30 or 60 minutes. The relevance of stress test results is significantly increased if for the sake of comparison a formulation is tested simultaneously for which long-term data at room temperature are available. The comparison with a "reference" in combination with experience gathered in the earlier phases of the stability testing which allows one to choose reasonable stress conditions is what makes the stress test predictions meaningful.

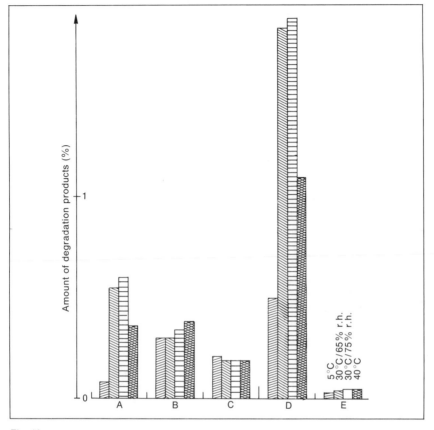

Fig. 10

A *comparative* stress test is recommended in the new FDA Guidelines (14), e. g. in the case of a galenical process change for a preparation already on the market. The same officials also recommend a stress test for ANDA's in the market packaging at 37–40 °C/75% R. H. for 1, 2 and 3 months (14). If results are satisfactory, a shelf-life of up to 24 months may be granted.

5. Stability of proposed product

The long-term stability test for the formulation which is intended for registration forms the heart of the entire stability testing procedure. The products must be tested in packaging which corresponds to the market packaging. Usually there are several types of packaging, first of all because it is seldom clear from the start which packaging affords optimal protection and cost advantages, and secondly because a single type of packaging is not sufficient for worldwide marketing of a medication. This testing in various packagings leads in particular to high costs because several batches must be tested (three as a rule).

To prevent a cost explosion, a certain degree of flexibility on the part of registration officials is desired so that, for instance, results in packaging A can be recognized for packaging B as long as the equivalency of the two packagings has been proven in a separate test. For tablets, for example, a change to packaging providing greater moisture protection is unproblematic. For liquid and semi-solid forms on the other hand, stability data from batches in the original container are normally absolutely necessary because interaction between packaging and contents is much stronger (15).

In recent years, the push through (or blister) packaging (PTP) for solid forms like tablets, coated tablets and capsules has become more and more successful in western Europe. Mainly transparent or opaque PVC is used as blister film which can be coated with PVDC (polyvinylidene chloride) or PCTFE (polychlorotrifluoroethylene) to increase protection against moisture. Along with the many advantages of the PTP, like customer appeal and protection of each unit until use, it has the disadvantage when compared to a glass packaging with a good stopper that less protection against moisture is afforded. Since the stability of solid forms usually deteriorates significantly when moisture is absorbed because, for example, hydrolysis reactions with the active ingredient proceed at an accelerated rate, this is a serious disadvantage.

Figure 11 shows the increase in weight of a PVC (250 µm)-PTP filled with silica gel tablets (a) and a PVC/PCTFE (200/19 µm)-PTP filled with tablets made of approx. 75% lactose and approx. 20% maize starch (b). All curves approximate a final value (first rapidly and then more and more slowly) which corresponds to the maximal water absorption of the preparation without packaging. The extra protection of the PVC/PCTFE film is very effective in the case of very high water absorption capacity (a). If only little water is absorbed, the effect of the more protective film is slight. The tablets (b) in fig. 11 are representative of many pharmaceutical preparations. For these types of product a good PVC/PCTFE-PTP provides good protection against moisture in *temperate* climates. In warm or tropical climates the protection is significantly reduced since the water vapor permeability of the film increases greatly as temperature increases. For effective protection against moisture in tropical climates the permeability of the films would have to be significantly lower than that of the best PVC/PCTFE films available today.

If the relationship between moisture in the surrounding air and absorption of water by the preparation, i.e. the sorption isotherm, and the permeability of the Push-Through-Package (PTP) are known, the water absorption can be calculated in advance. Figure 12 shows a computer simulation of this type. It was assumed that the sorption isotherm is linear, which is largely speaking true for most preparations below a critical moisture limit, and that the diffusion of water vapor through the film

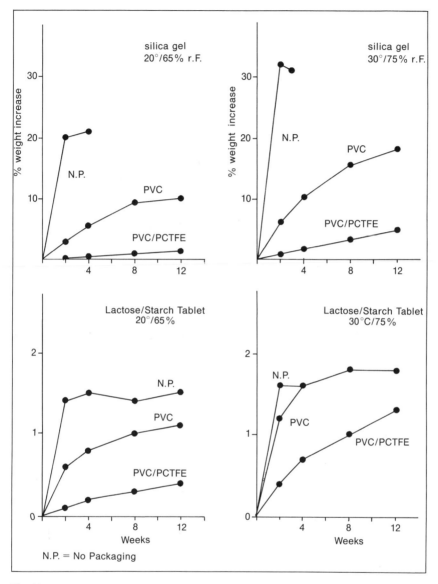

Fig. 11

could be described by Fick's 1st law. The following typical values were assumed for the permeability of the (molded!) blister films:

PVC: 20 °C: 40 m Perm
            30 °C: 60 m Perm

PVC/PCTFE: 20 °C: 4 m Perm
            30 °C: 8 m Perm

The large difference in protection offered by the films at 20°C/65% R.H. can clearly be seen as well as the reduction of this protection as water absorption capacity of the product decreases and the short protection period at 30°C/75%, even with the least permeable film. These relationships are taken into consideration when selecting the packaging in which the stability of a product is to be tested.

For worldwide marketing of a medication, the test must be carried out at several temperatures and humidities corresponding to various climate zones. The test conditions are not internationally standardized. An example of a test plan for solid forms is given in fig. 13. The results at 25°C/50% R.H. are valid for temperature and Mediterranean-like climates, those at 30°C/65% for warm climate zones and those at 30°C/75% for tropical zones. The samples stored at − 25°C serve solely as the reference for the chemical testing. The results at 40°C are used to compare batches and to evaluate transport hazards. Testing at 50°C is required by law in some countries.

This test plan provides sufficient data for registration in almost all countries. The most important exception is the Japanese registration guidelines, which stipulate among other things (for all products with normal stability) that in every case a test at room temperature over 3 years must be performed ("Method A"). Since "room temperature" is not exactly defined as it is for us, but is rather supposed to encompass

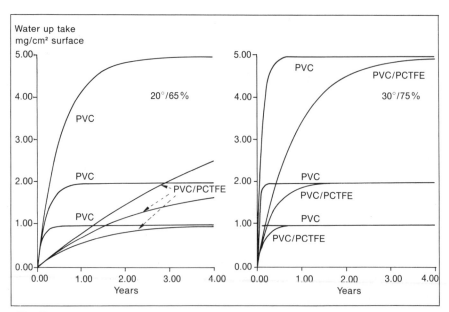

Fig. 12

all the climatic conditions prevailing in Japan at the time including all of the seasonal fluctuations, in practice there is no alternative but to perform or repeat this test in Japan itself. It is not specified in which geographical region of Japan the test must occur: the warm southern part or the rather cold North. Considering the flexibility allowed within the country itself, this drastic confinement to the Japanese borders cannot be supported scientifically and it is ununderstandable why stability tests performed under controlled conditions in other countries should then not also be acceptable. It is imperative to demand that this type of one-sided technical registration limitation be dropped in favor of a flexible attitude on the part of officials toward non-national producers.

A certain amount of flexibility should also be shown with respect to the testing sequence. This would make it possible, for example, to test several batches simultaneously, which would significantly reduce analysis costs since rationalization measures in collecting samples for analysis series are very effective. Seldom can the stability batches be produced and stored in the climatic rooms at such ideal time intervals that by adhering to rigid analysis schedules the analysis dates of different batches coincide, for example, the 36-month samples from the first batch with the 24-month samples from the second batch. By exercising some flexibility with the time schedule, especially in the second year and on in the long-term test, this cost reduction could be achieved without adversely affecting the batch comparison, as will be shown.

By collecting batches for testing, not only are the costs reduced, but the precision and reliability of the data is increased because the apparatus settings, reagents and the analyst's technique are constant. This so-called "gang stability program" has been very successfully used for stability monitoring of products already on the market (16) and no scientific grounds exist which speak against implementing this

Figure 13: Stability Testing Protocol for solid dosage forms for world-wide marketing

Packaging	G	BG	BG	B	BG	G
Conditions Time (months)	−25°C	25°C 50% R.H.	30°C 65% R.H.	30°C 75% R.H.	40°C	50°C
0		CP				
3	C	CP	CP	CP	CP	CP
6	C	CP	CP	CP	CP	CP
12	C	CP	CP	CP		
24	C	CP	CP	CP		
36	C	CP	CP	CP		
48	C	CP	CP			
60	C	CP	CP			

Notes: G = Glass   C = Chemical testing
        B = Blister   P = Physical testing

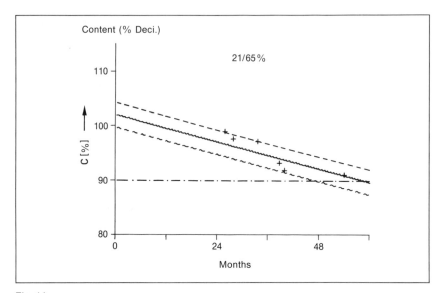

Fig. 14

concept in the later phases of the long-term testing during development, from the second year on, for example. If one analyses the data graphically and/or with mathematical models, e.g. regression calculation, the batch comparison can be performed just as well as if each batch had been analysed according to a fixed schedule. Figure 14 demonstrates the evaluation of a stability trial according to this principle. The contents of intact active ingredient is shown. The data were evaluated using linear regression. Since only differences in the *stability* are tested here, the differences in initial values for the batches (which are not relevant in this respect) were mathematically eliminated. (All data were converted to percentages of the average of the initial contents values for all batches.)

In fig. 14 the resulting regression calculation and confidence limits for the individual values (P = 95%, one-sided) are represented. One can see immediately that these batches are quite homogeneous. This is confirmed by the residual variance which is a measue of the residual scatter not explainable by the regression calculation. The root of the residual variance cannot be less than the coefficient of variation (= relative standard deviation) of the applied analytical method. In our example the root of the residual variance is 1.25%, which is not significantly larger than the coefficient of variation for the HPLC method which was used (1%). Therefore, no indication is given that an outlier with respect to stability is among the batches examined. Even this simple calculation allows us to make a batch comparison which is at least as good as if all batches had been analysed according to a strict schedule. The quality of the comparison is even better because of the low scatter of the data. More extensive statistical evaluations, like an F-test, are possible (9), (16); however, in the example they provide no further information.

6. Conclusion

In this short overview, which necessarily must remain incomplete, it was tried, using examples, to shed light on some of the problems which can arise in stability testing during preparation development. Stability testing is a continuous process which generates more and more knowledge. Information on the drug substance and the first provisional dosage forms is synergistic and builds the basis for the development of the dosage form which will be marketed. The successful coordination of short- and long-term trials is of decisive importance. The test conditions must be suited to the product being tested. Registration guidelines should specify the type of information to be provided – the "what" – but allow enough freedom in the question of "how", i. e. the test plans (storage conditions: temperature, moisture, test frequency), at least until harmonization of such guidelines has been achieved on the international level.

Literatur

(1) PMA's joint QC-PDS Stability Committee, "Stability Concepts" Pharmaceutical Technology, June 1984
(2) Witthaus, G., in "Topics in Pharmaceutical Sciences", Ed. D. Breimer and P. Speiser, Elsevier 1981, p. 275
(3) Leuenberger H., Becher W., Pharm. Acta Helv. 50, 88 (1975)
(4) El-Shattawy H. H., Drug Dev. Ind. Pharm. 8, 819 (1982)
(5) Dukes G. R., Drug. Dev. Ind. Pharm. 10, 1413 (1984)
(6) Ondracek, J., Boller, F. H., Zullinger, H. W., Niederer, R. R., Acta Pharm. Techn. 31, 42 (1985)
(7) Grimm W., Schepky G., Stabilitätsprüfung in der Pharmazie, Editio Cantor Aulendorf (1980)
(8) Thoma K., Arzneimittelstabilität, Werbe- und Vertriebsgesellschaft Deutscher Apotheker mbH, Frankfurt/Main (1978)
(9) Hartmann V., Bethke H., Michaelis W., Krummen K. and Baltzer M. O. in "Pharmazeutische Qualitätskontrolle" Ed. H. Feltkamp, P. Fuchs and H. Sucker, Georg Thieme Verlag, Stuttgart, New York, 1983 p. 524
(10) Kersten D., Göber B., Die Pharmazie, 39, 213 (1984)
(11) Hoblitzel J. R., Thakker K. D., Rhodes C. T., Pharm. Acta Helv. 60, 28 (1985)
(12) Rudnic E. M., Lausier J. M., Rhodes C. T., Drug Dev. Ind. Pharm. 5, 589 (1979)
(13) Molokhia A. M., Moustafa M. A., Gouda M. W., Drug Dev. Ind. Pharm. 8, 283 (1982)
(14) Draft Guideline for Stability Studies for Human Drugs and Biologics, FDA, August 1985
(15) Davies J. S., Drug Dev. Ind. Pharm. 10, 1549 (1984)
(16) Thompson, K., Drug Dev. Ind. Pharm. 10, 1449 (1984)

XVII. Packaging materials and shelf-life

D. Herrmann, Schering AG, Berlin

1. Introduction/General remarks

As a rule, drug formulations are mixtures of physically and chemically reactive substances. They are often impaired in their shelf-life by the action of external influences, e. g., as a result of the absorption of water vapour from a moist atmosphere or oxidation caused by the oxygen in the air. Light can lead to photochemical decomposition. Other drug formulations are inclined to dry out, e. g., alcoholic solutions and tinctures or also aqueous formulations. Not only solutions but also lotions and creams are hazarded. It is only through the selection of suitable packaging materials that satisfactory shelf-life can be attained in such cases. It may also be said that the microclimate which is best for shelf-life must be ensured inside the package.

The packaging material itself is, likewise, subject to changes caused by climatic influences. Its shelf-life must be markedly superior to that of its contents. On the other hand, the packaging material must be inert in relation to its contents; it should therefore neither release nor absorb substances.

These are indeed absolute demands which have to be relativized for practical requirements. Just as protection from external influences cannot be total, the requirement of inertness must be restricted to a standard which can be classified as safe or harmless.

Considered in its totality, we therefore have a threecornered relationship: drug formulation – packaging material – environmental influences. As part of the selection of packaging materials, the individual aspects must be assessed in relation to each other in each case and also in relation to the shelf-life of the drug product in its entirety.

In the course of the development of a new drug preparation, the selection and suitability testing of packaging materials is usually arranged at a point in time between the selection studies for establishing the most suitable formulation and the long-term stability test. It would be very expensive to multiply the number of investigational series for establishing the formulation by the number of all the alternative packaging materials which could be considered. On the other hand, it is desirable to start the long-term stability test of the so-called "final formulation" in the "final container" at the earliest date possible. This is why use has to be made of stress tests. Other bases are the knowledge of the physical and chemical properties of the drug formulation observed in the course of establishing the drug formulation and

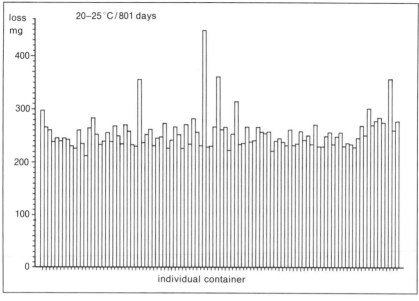

Fig. 1

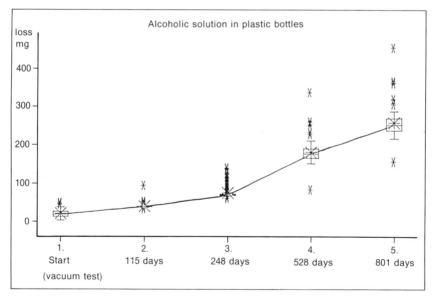

Fig. 2

general experience. The selection of packaging materials is therefore of a markedly prognostic character. The prognosis must then be confirmed in the long term. In the event of instability, an attempt must be made to identify the cause so that knowledge of the subject can be updated.

2. Permeation/Plastic bottles

It is often the case that delimitation of the various factors affecting the stability of the drug formulation is only possible through the application of statistical methods, e. g., the distinction between the tightness of a plastic bottle in the closure area and the permeation of the solvent through the wall-material. Of course, the tightness of the closure is one of the basic demands. Stability testing of objects known to leak is obviously a waste of time. In the example shown, however, it is a question of micro-leakages which remain unnoticed in a normal leakage test and only become obvious in the course of several months. The subsequent loosening of sorew-caps or the opening of seals or adhesive closures under the influence of the pharmaceutical preparation must be considered. And as regards the permeability of the packaging materials, it is quite possible for this to change in the course of storage, e. g., as a result of swelling.

Fig. 1 shows a histogram which illustrates the loss by evaporation of individual bottles containing an alcoholic solution in a group of uniform bottles of high-density polyethylene. In some cases, the different bar-lengths show quite considerable losses by evaporation from individual objects whereas, otherwise, it is a question of scatter of a much lower order.

The histogram was drawn with the aid of a plotter after the input of the data. The follow-up program used calculates the arithmetical mean and the median value and presents these in graph form within the range of the 25–75% quantiles (Fig. 2). The values outside this quantile area are represented as bars up to the single box-plot length. These bar-lengths, with an adequate approximation, comprise the 95% confidence range of a Gaussian distribution. Values outside this are shown individually. They can be regarded as mavericks. Only by means of microscopic investigations it can be decided whether the mavericks are caused by microleaks in the closure area or by anomal wall-thickness or other defects. But such investigations are destructive and the bottles cannot be stored any longer. It is now possible to eliminate the mavericks from the data-files and to restart the program. It was decided not to do this since the number of bottles with micro-leaks or other defects remained the same and the influence on the position of the mean value was only slight.

Fig. 3 shows the average loss by evaporation. The median value, the maximum value and the minimum value are plotted against the duration of the test. The rise-rate of the median value is of satisfactory uniformity and justifies the extrapolation to a longer duration of time. The permeability through the wall-material has obviously not changed. No serious deterioration in the closure tightness has occured either. The diagrams are all based on storage in a normal climate. It is self-evident that the results of storage-tests carried out in parallel under other test-climates are also to be considered in the conclusions drawn in respect of the suitability of the container in question for the preparation. This example apart from the differention between the evaporation routes, also clearly shows the differences existing between the individual objects.

3. Lyophilisates/Freeze-drying stoppers

In special cases, an active influence by the packaging material on the water content of drug formulations must also be reckoned with. Lyophilisates are usually extremely hygroscopic and, as a possible source of an increased water content in the course of storage, consideration must also be given to the stopper material.

For the comparative investigation of the water content of stoppers, use can be made of the determination of the water vapour released at 180 °C in a stream of pre-dried nitrogen by coulometric indication (Fig. 4). From this, it is apparent that the normal drying of stoppers is not very effective. Only a specific vacuum-drying effects an adequate reduction in the water content of the stoppers for special purposes.

Further conclusions are possible: Initially a rapid rise in the quantity of coulometrically measured water vapour is observed. This is presumably water which is adsorbed to the surface of the stopper. Later a protracted diffusion process becomes established; this is attributed to the release of moisture from the interior of the stopper.

4. Glass

With this example of the release of moisture from freeze-drying stoppers we can move from the purely protective effect in the sense of the "preservation of tightness/limitation of permeation" to interaction due to the release of substances from the packaging material. The group of packaging materials known as "glass" supplies several pertinent exemples.

The subdivision of glass-types according to the European-Pharmacopeia is well known. First of all, a distinction is drawn between soda-lime glass, Type III glass, and neutral glass, Type I glass. Type III glass can be annealed to obtain Type II glass. There is no difference between glass of Type I and II in respect of the alkali which is transferred from them to an aqueous solution stored in a bottle. This is what is of primary interest to the pharmacist. According to their suitability, glass of both Type I and Type II may equally be used for aqueous parenteral solutions. This reservation of

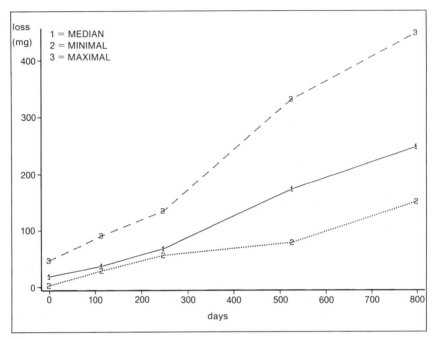

Fig. 3

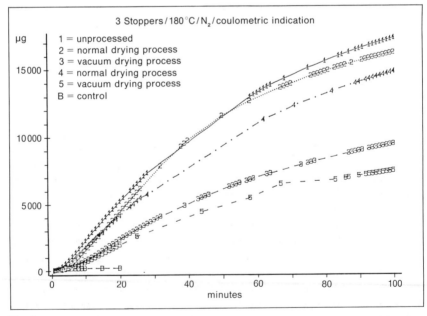

Fig. 4

Table 1: Typical glass compositions

| | Type I glass | | | | Type III glass | |
| | tubular glass | | molded glass | | molded glass | |
	colourless	brown	colourless	brown	colourless	brown
SiO_2	74.6	72.0	71.1	66.2	72.0	72.0
Al_2O_3	4.6	5.0	4.6	6.6	2.0	2.2
B_2O_3	10.0	9.0	11.5	8.6	0.6	0.6
Na_2O	6.3	6.0	8.3	8.1	13.5	14.0
K_2O	–	1.0	0.7	1.1	0.4	0.4
CaO	0.5	1.0	1.36	0.7	9.0	9.2
MgO	–	–	–	–	2.5	1.0
BaO	3.9	2.0	2.42	1.2	–	0.4
Fe_2O_3	<0.05	1.0	<0.05	0.1	–	0.2
TiO_2	–	3.0	–	–	–	–
MnO	–	–	–	6.0	–	–

Review according: S.V. Sanga, Bull. parent. drug. ass. Vol. 33 No. 2 (1979) 61–67

suitability is made in the USP XXI for alkaline formulations and takes account of the actual facts. The annealing layer is very thin, thinner than 1 μm and can be dissolved by alkaline solutions. The mere fulfillment of a pharmacopeial requirement, in this case the fulfillment of the alkali limit requirement, is not sufficient. The actual suitability must be assured by stability tests.

What do the types of glass really imply and what conclusions can be drawn from them? A quality grading is usually inferred from the glass designation sequence of Type I, II and III. However, it is not a question of quality gradings but of different identities. II and I can be equivalent and in certain cases II can even be superior to I. This is so, for example, with largevolume infusion bottles.

Table 1 shows typical compositions of various types of glass. Glass can be defined as the undercooled melt of silicic acid and metal oxides. This is why it is usual to list metal oxides, irrespective of the true chemical bond.

In Type I glass, there is a higher proportion of boron and aluminium than in normal soda-lime glass. This effects the large reduction in the release of alkali by Type I glass. But Type II glass is very different. During the annealing process of soda-lime glass, alkali and alkaline earths are extracted. A thin layer resembling quartz glass is left, since this glass has a low level of other components. This layer can be destroyed, e. g., by an alkaline solution's being filled into the bottle. In special cases, e. g., with solutions which are particularly rich in sodium ions, a re-absorption of sodium ions is possible. The previously greatly shrunk and thus compacted layer of quartz glass swells, allowing alkali to be diffused from the deeper layers of glass in the direction of the aqueous solutions filled into the bottle.

From the above remarks, it could be inferred, that Type I glass is less complicated. But there are other risks. Type I glass is only characterized by a particularly low alkali release when it has not been overheated. When the glass is shaped into ampoules and especially injection vials, it is possible that glass condensates are generated. These condensates release considerable amounts of alkali. The quantity of alkali can vary greatly from one injection vial to another. This possibility must be considered in the assessment of the results of long-term stability tests. For example, this might be a simple explanation for differences in the pH-values of a pharmaceutical preparation measured in individual ampoules or vials.

The powdered glass test which is used to distinguish between Type I glass and soda-lime glass is not able to detect this deterioration in quality. This can only be revealed by the surface methods. It should be noted that the limit value definition for the amount of alkali released from the inner surface of the containers refers to the mean value, either by pooling of the contents of individual containers for the titration or by averaging individual test results obtained by atomic absorption.

The components of glass are divided into exchangeable components and components of low exchangeability. Alkali and alkaline earths belong to the first group, the exchangeable components, while the second group includes not only boron and aluminium but also iron and manganese. The latter elements, iron and manganese, are pigments of brown glasses. Even under drastic conditions, iron ions are scarcely released from brown glasses – the Japanese Pharmacopeia gives such a specification – and in normal circumstances do not endanger the stability of pharmaceutical solutions. Apart from the low solubility, one would endeavour anyway to stabilize an active agent endangered by heavy metal catalysis by the addition of complexing agents to the pharmaceutical solution. When the qualitative and quantitative compositions of colourless glasses are considered in comparison with brown glasses, it will be found that all the brown glasses have additionally nothing but the pigment components. It should therefore be legitimate to apply stability experience obtained from storage tests in brown glasses to colourless glasses and vice versa if a sufficient number of representative tests have been carried out to ensure equivalence. Similarly, the usability of non-annealed soda-lime glass implies the usability of annealed glass, likewise subject to proof by evidence.

5. Light protection

For the evaluation of the light-protective effect of brown glasses and other packaging materials, special attention should be paid to the short-wave part of the spectrum. It is this part in particular which is photochemically active. Most pharmacopeias consequently specify that the transmission of light be measured in the 290–450 nm range. Lower wavelengths do not need to be considered since they are not present in normal daylight. And indeed it should be self-evident that bright sunlight must always be kept away from drug formulations, even when these are not declared as sensitive to light.

If the absorption curves of various brown glasses are considered, it will be noticed

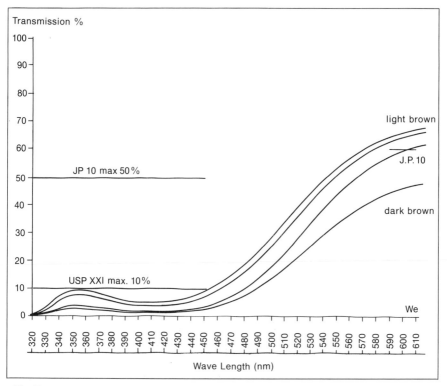

Fig. 5

that there is a residual transmission in the photochemically active range and that this is also tolerated by the pharmacopeias (Fig. 5). A glass which is almost completely absorbent in this range would not be transparent enough to allow a visual check to be made, for example, for foreign particles in a solution for parenteral use. The light-protective effect of coloured primary packaging materials cannot therefore be complete and an additional label "Store protected from light" will be necessary. The extent to which this is realized by the dispensing pharmacist, prescribing physician or the patient, since brown glass certainly suggests full protection from light, cannot be assessed.

While the majority of pharmacopeias only describe the colour of glass in general terms, the Japanese and also the Korean Pharmacopeia specify minimum transparency values. The limitvalue specification is for 600 nm, i.e., outside of the photochemically active range. In actual fact, this minimum value is met only by light-brown or honey-coloured glass. Consequently, these pharmacopeias also permit a higher transmission of light in the photochemically active range and therefore accept a reduced light-protective effect. This is without doubt a compromise to assist the recognition of particles and fibers.

According to the European Pharmacopeia, brown glass should not be used for formulations with a tendency to discolour. This, too, is obviously based on the need for a visual check of the contents. The fact that variations in the colour of pharmaceutical solutions, as can occur during storage, cannot be a suitable criterion of quality for the dispensing pharmacist or the attending doctor since these do not have access to the appropriate reference standards, is only mentioned in passing and is not in opposition to this requirement.

Also according to the European Pharmacopeia, brown glass may only be used for extremely sensitive pharmaceutical solutions. The term "extreme sensitivity to light" is not specifically defined and this is also not necessary. A formulation cannot really be classed as extremely sensitive to light if damage caused to it by exposure to light only becomes manifest after several hours' exposure. The usual statement refers to 600 lux. This is equivalent to the brightness at a normal working-position. When it is a question of higher light-intensities, the exposure time which can be tolerated is reduced accordingly. It is selfevident that protection from light by the secondary packaging material, i.e., by the outer box, must also be ensured for preparations which are only moderately sensitive to light. However, as already mentioned, this also applies to brown glass.

6. Elastomers/Rubber materials

Since even the glass is of such importance in the assessment, what is the effect then of rubber parts and what influence do they have on the stability of drug formulations? Rubber parts, also designated as elastomers, are in general regarded as very complex materials. Nevertheless, it should be possible, at least for internal use, to establish categories similar to those used for glass, within which analogy conclusions are permissible in respect of stability.

It is customary to divide rubber materials into those which are sulphur cured and those not containing sulphur. This definition is not very satisfactory since there are additives containing sulphur for modern non-conventionally cross-linked elastomers, but it at least endeavours to make a basic distinction. For the vulcanization of natural rubber, for example, use is made of sulphur and so-called vulcanization accelerators. These are substances with a certain solubility in water which can impair the stability of drug formulations. And, apart from sulphates, sulphur compounds are well-known for their numerous interactions.

This concerns not only natural rubbers but also conventionally cross-linked nitrile and butyl rubbers for which accelerators are likewise used. In contrast to this, modern halobutyl rubbers do not need such additives. The actual cross-linking takes place without the use of sulphur and activation is achieved by zinc oxide or magnesium oxide, substances which are also employed for conventionally vulcanized parts. As a positive consequence of the omission of sulphur and accelerator substances, scarcely any chemical extractive substances are found in the usual autoclave tests of halobutyl rubbers.

For the testing of the amount of extractive substances released, 200 ml of water for injection are poured over rubber parts with a defined surface, e. g., three infusion stoppers with a total area of 100 cm². The flask is closed in a suitable manner and autoclaved in the steam sterilizer. The usual steam sterilization of pharmaceutical solutions is thus simulated. After cooling, the aqueous extract solution is decanted and is available for the tests (table 2). In the case of conventionally vulcanized materials, considerable quantitaties of reducing substances are found. This value is expressed in terms of consumption of potassium permanganate and is determined by titration. In addition, the non volatile residue and the u/v absorbance are also of interest. By contrast, the criteria in question are about 0 in each case for halobutyl rubber.

Table 2: Rubber Test Results

Chemical safety Test-No. a) 838/8 b) V 1345	Berlin, 14.12.71/07.07.81		SCHERING Pharmaceutical Laboratory
Description: Infusion stopper a) red b) black Supplier: A B Designation:			
Material identification: a) natural rubber, containing sulphur b) chlorobutylrubber, sulphur-free			
Results of tests according to Pharm. Lab. Spec. M6/DIN 58367 Shore hardness: a) 48 b) 49 Vol. sulphides: a) negative b) negative Ash content: a) 32% b) 3.7% Extraction test: (3 samples/200 ml water 30 mins. 121°C) Sample:	a) Result	b)	Requirement:
Description of autocl. material:	unchanged	unchanged	unchanged
Description of test-solution:	slightly turbid rubber smell	clear odourless	clear to opalescent colourless
Ammonium:	still permissible	negative	max. 0.02 mg/10 ml
Chloride:	negative	negative	max. 0.04 mg/10 ml
Heavy metals:	negative	negative	max. 0.01 mg Pb^{++}/10 ml
Zinc:	negative	negative	max. 0.03 mg/10 ml
pH test solution pH comparison	7.6 6.5	6.6 6.3	shift max. 1 pH-unit

Continue Tab. 2

Reduc. components				
	0.8		approx. 0	max. 1.5 ml 0.01 N KMnO$_4$
Dry residue:	2.4		approx. 0	max. 4 mg/100 ml
U/V$_{absorbance}$	E$_{1 cm}$			
320 nm	1.22	0		
310 nm	0.965			
300 nm	0.524			
290 nm	0.326			
280 nm	0.308			
270 nm	0.274	} < 0.1		
260 nm	0.396			
250 nm	0.510			
240 nm	0.786			
230 nm	1.103			
220 nm	1.177			
210 nm	1.670	0.1		
Remarks:	a) polyisoprene conventionally vulcanized filler CaCO$_3$		b) halobutyl rubber unconventionally cross-linked filler carbon black	

Substances with an extraction capability of this nature are a potential burden for the stability of pharmaceutical solutions. Even though the chemical identity of the individual elastomer additives probably varies to a considerable extent, a relation between the amount of substances released from the stopper and the chemical stability of the pharmaceutical solution is often noted in comparative stability tests, ranging, for example, from conventionally sulphur-cured butyl rubber via conventional natural rubber to the practically inert halobutyl and silicone rubbers. Account must naturally be taken of the intrinsic decomposition characteristics of the solution when stored for several months under the same test conditions. Experience has shown that lacquers are not able to control interactions to a desirable extent; they are used, or were formerly used, mainly from the aspect of reducing the release of particulate matter.

Another group to which the elastomers can be assigned is their permeability to gases and vapours. Without regard to the chemical properties just discussed above, the high-density butyl and halobutyl rubbers are to be grouped together in contrast to the natural rubbers and synthetic isoprene. The latter group displays higher permeation rates and should therefore be avoided where possible for pharmaceutical formulations which are especially endangered. In keeping with this increased permeability to gases and vapours, low-dosage substances in pharmaceutical solutions tend to be absorbed by such elastomers. This applies to preservatives, for example. In comparison, the high-density butyl and halobutyl rubbers display less absorption.

A third group could concern the loading or filler system, e. g., certain fillers cause recrystallization phenomens. As an example, barium sulphate may be mentioned. It recrystallizes without a chemical reaction. Calcium carbonate can form salts of poor solubility with components of the pharmaceutical solution and in this manner can, likewise, induce turbidity.

7. Plastic/General categories

This suffices for the area of the elastomers. In the areas of plastics, it is easier to form groups within which analogy conclusions can be drawn with respect to stability of the pharmaceutical preparation. PVC foils may be considered. These are usually similar to each other in respect of water-vapour permeation which is the determining factor for their use as blister strips for coated and uncoated tablets. Polyethylenes, likewise, form self-contained groups whereby a distinction is to be drawn between high-density and low-density polyethylene. By reason of similar physical properties and similar additive selection, high-density polyethylene can be classed with polypropylene.

8. Collapsible tubes/Aluminium

Finally, metal tubes should also be briefly discussed. Depending on the acid strength of the preparation with which they are filled, corrosion of the aluminium can occur. The swelling due to the development of gas and the appearance of holes as a result of the metal being dissolved by the contents are well known. The use of protective lacquers is therefore customary; epoxy resin lacquers are preferred. After stoving, these lacquers are very resistant and are largely free from chemical interactions with the contents of the tube. However, this protective effect presupposes adequate lacquering of the entire inner area. Inadequately lacquered spots can be detected with the aid of the sublimate test. After brief contact with a mercury chloride solution, efflorescences appear at inadequately protected spots. This is without doubt a basic requirement; there is just as little point in carrying out long-term stability tests with faulty tubes as there is with leaky bottles. Within the framework of a series of stability tests, we observed special interactions between the metal of the tube and its contents. Thorough examination revealed in each case a noticeable reduction in the lacquer coating at the mouth of the tube. Without doubt, this is a consequence of the lacquering technique. To this extent, it may be compared with the example of micro-leaks in bottles containing an alcoholic solution mentioned at the beginning of this paper.

9. Conclusions/Summery

To sum up, it follows that prognoses can be made in respect of suitability from the aspect of stability optimization in the assessment of packaging materials. The appropriate compilation of stability rest results permits individual groups of packaging materials to be established, within which conclusions based on analogy are possible.